Natural Remedies & Herbal Healing A Beginner's Guide

Discover the Power of Nature: Enhance Your Well-being with Herbs and Natural Remedies

Tammy Andrews

Table of Contents

CHAPTER 6
HERBS AROMATIC

Introduction

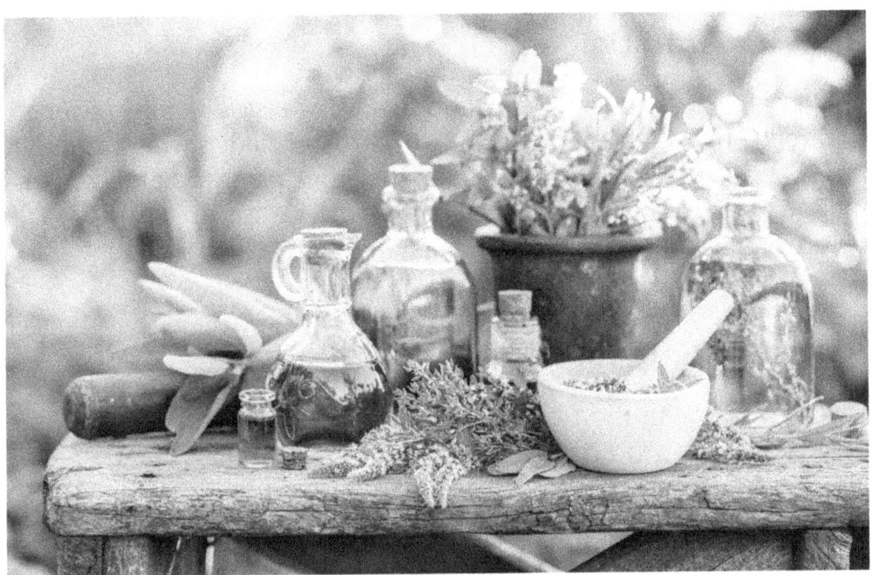

Welcome to "A Beginner's Guide: Natural Remedies & Herbal Healing." In the fast-paced world we live in, the allure of natural remedies and herbal healing has captivated many seeking alternatives to conventional approaches. This guide serves as a gateway for those embarking on a journey into the world of herbal wellness. Discover the Power of Nature

Nature has been our original pharmacy, offering a myriad of remedies for various ailments. In this guide, we will explore the timeless wisdom of herbal healing, uncovering the potential of plants to enhance our well-being. Whether you are new to the concept or seeking to deepen your understanding, this guide is crafted with beginners in mind, providing a solid foundation for your exploration.

Navigating the Chapters

The chapters unfold like a map, guiding you through essential aspects of natural remedies and herbal healing. From the historical roots of herbalism to the practical application of herbs in daily life, each section is tailored to empower you with knowledge and practical insights.

Bridging Tradition and Science

We'll bridge the gap between traditional wisdom and modern science, unraveling the historical significance of herbal remedies while exploring the scientific principles that validate their effectiveness. Safety is paramount, and we encourage you to consult with healthcare professionals before embarking on any new herbal regimen.

Herbal Healing for Common Ailments

Discover how common herbs can become your allies in addressing everyday health concerns. We'll delve into combinations, preparations, and the safe integration of herbs into your daily routine, ensuring a holistic approach to your well-being.

Your Personal Herbal Journey

Whether you're seeking relief from specific conditions or aiming for general well-being, this guide invites you to embark on a personal herbal journey. It is not just a book; it's a companion for those eager to unlock the potential of natural remedies.

Empower Yourself

As you navigate through these pages, empower yourself with knowledge that transcends generations. Natural remedies and herbal healing are not just practices; they are invitations to reconnect with the healing power of nature.

So, welcome to the beginning of your herbal adventure. May this guide serve as your compass, leading you toward a harmonious and empowered relationship with the world of natural remedies and herbal healing.

CHAPTER 1

The World of Healing Herbs

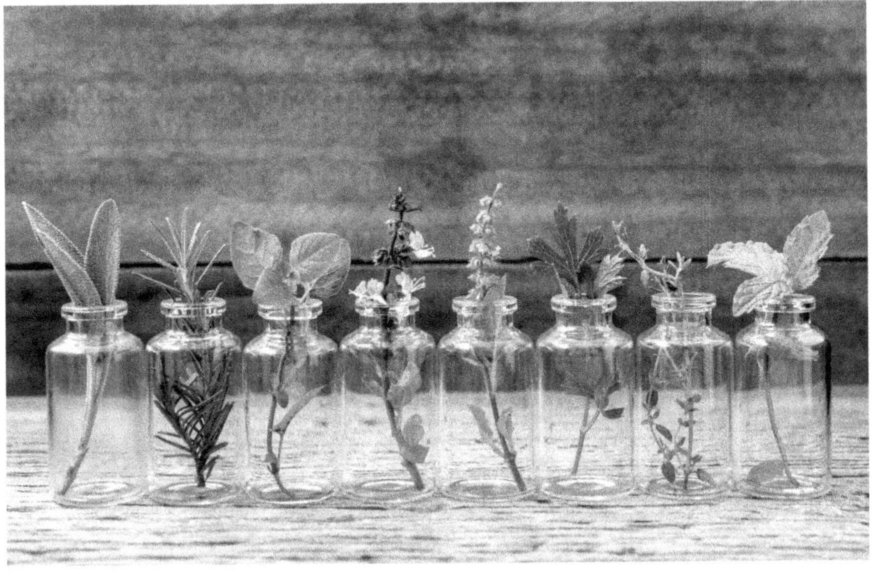

Herbs, ancient custodians of natural wisdom, unveil their mysterious potential in the art of self-healing. Embodying knowledge passed down through centuries and cultures, these plants offer a unique blend of ancient traditions and modern science. On one hand, they transport us back in time, immersing us in the rich herbal traditions from every corner of the globe. On the other, they unveil their biochemical complexity, revealing a natural pharmacy rich in active compounds. Identifying, harvesting, and preserving these botanical wonders becomes a ritual that marries respect for the earth with the care of the body and mind. Herbs, with their aromatic and healing nuances, become precious allies in our quest for balance and well-being. Exploring their world is an invitation to reconnect with nature and discover a treasure trove of solutions for health, sourced from the very earth that nurtures us.

Ancient Traditions and Modern Herbal Science

At the heart of our guide, we delve into the world of healing herbs—a realm that has fascinated humanity throughout the ages. We will explore the ancient herbal traditions that have shaped our relationship with plants, not neglecting the intriguing intersection with modern herbal science.

Herbs in Different Cultures

Every culture has its rich history of herbalism. From Ayurveda to Chinese herbalism, we will delve into specific traditions that have influenced herbal usage worldwide.

Convergence of Tradition and Scientific Research

We will discover how traditional herbal practices align with modern scientific discoveries, creating a synergy that values the best of both worlds. Research continues to unveil the biochemical secrets of plants, affirming the value of ancient herbal wisdom.

Identification, Harvesting, and Preservation of Herbs

Identifying Herbs

Properly identifying herbs is crucial to ensure their effectiveness and safety. We will explore practical methods to recognize plants, analyzing leaves, flowers, and distinctive features.

Responsible Harvesting

A practical guide to responsibly harvesting herbs. We will discuss the ideal times for harvesting, usable plant parts, and sustainable practices to preserve biodiversity.

Preserving Herb Properties

Once harvested, it is essential to properly preserve herbs to maintain their therapeutic properties. We will explore drying methods, storage, and preparation for future use.

Active Compounds and Benefits of Herbs

Bioactive Substances

Herbs contain a vast range of bioactive substances responsible for their beneficial effects. From vitamins to flavonoids, we will analyze these key substances and their impact on human health.

Therapeutic Properties of Common Herbs

A detailed list of the therapeutic properties of the most common herbs. From chamomile to lavender, we will discover how these plants can contribute to our overall well-being.

Preparation and Practical Use of Herbs

Infusions, Decoctions, and Tinctures

A detailed analysis of different preparation methods, from creating infusions and decoctions to the tincturing process. Each method will have its focus, ensuring you can choose the one most suitable for your needs.

Herbal Culinary Arts

We will explore how to integrate herbs into your daily cuisine, not just for taste but also for health benefits. Recipes and tips to make cooking a herbal experience.

Herbs in Treating Common Ailments

Pain and Inflammation

We will explore herbs that can contribute to relieving pain and inflammation, providing natural alternatives to conventional medications.

Stress and Anxiety

Herbs suitable for managing stress and anxiety, offering natural support for mental well-being.

Safety and Side Effects

Precautions

An in-depth discussion of precautions to take when using herbs, especially for specific categories of people, such as pregnant women and individuals with pre-existing medical conditions.

Potential Side Effects

Detailed information on potential side effects of herbs, offering a balanced perspective on safety and effectiveness.

Integrating Herbs into Daily Life

Wellness Rituals

Practical suggestions on how to integrate herbs into your daily routine, creating small rituals that support your overall well-being.

Herbs for Beauty

We will discover how certain herbs can be used to promote beauty and skincare naturally.

In-Depth Insights on Herbs for Specific Conditions

Herbs for Sleep

A detailed guide to herbs that can promote restful and relaxing sleep.

Herbs for Digestive Health

How some herbs can support digestive health, addressing common issues such as indigestion and bloating.

Resources and References

Books, Websites, and Organizations

A comprehensive list of resources to continue your learning journey on healing herbs.

Concluding the Herbal Journey

We are only at the beginning of our journey into the world of healing herbs. We conclude this chapter by inviting you to explore further, experiment with curiosity, and embrace the transformative power of herbs in your everyday life.

CHAPTER 2

Herbs for Physical Well-Being

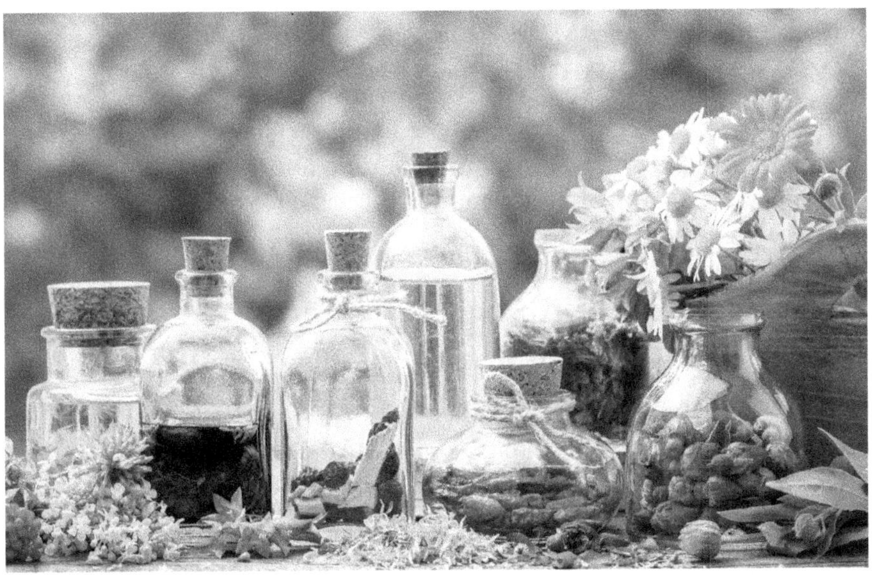

Introduction

In the vast world of herbs, we discover their crucial role in promoting physical well-being. These plants, rich in healing properties, become valuable allies on our journey towards optimal physical health.

Alleviating Pain with Anti-Inflammatory Herbs

Anti-inflammatory herbs such as turmeric, ginger, and boswellia can be used to manage chronic pain and reduce inflammation. Explore how these herbs can be utilized to enhance joint and muscle health.

Natural Energy with Adaptogenic Herbs

Adaptogenic herbs like ashwagandha and rhodiola stand out for their adaptability to stress and fatigue. Explore how these plants can increase physical endurance, reduce fatigue, and promote a healthy energy balance.

Boosting the Immune System

Immunostimulant herbs like echinacea and astragalus are crucial allies in supporting the immune system. Examine how these herbs can help prevent colds and flu, providing natural support for our immune health.

Detoxification and Body Cleansing

Herbs play an essential role in body detoxification. Explore the use of herbs such as milk thistle and dandelion leaves to support the liver and purify the blood, promoting the health of vital organs.

Improving Sleep Quality with Relaxing Herbs

Relaxing herbs like chamomile, valerian, and lemon balm can promote deep and quality sleep. Discover how to integrate these herbs into your evening routine to enhance nightly rest and support physical recovery.

Supporting Cardiovascular Health

Herbs like garlic, olive leaf, and hawthorn are associated with promoting cardiovascular health. Analyze how these plants can contribute to maintaining blood pressure and cholesterol levels.

Herbs for Joint and Bone Health

For those dealing with joint and bone issues, herbs like nettle, sage, and cherry plum can offer natural relief. Explore how these herbs can contribute to joint health and prevent conditions such as arthritis.

Hormonal Balance with Herbs

Certain herbs, such as maca root and licorice, are known for their positive impact on hormonal balance. Explore how these plants can be useful during life stages like menopause or to address occasional hormonal imbalances.

Conclusions

This chapter has provided an overview of herbs for physical well-being. The anti-inflammatory, immunostimulant, and relaxing properties of these herbs offer a natural approach to physical health. In the next chapter, we will delve further into the expansive world of herbs within the context of holistic well-being.

CHAPTER 3

Exploring the Profound Beneficial Properties of Herbs

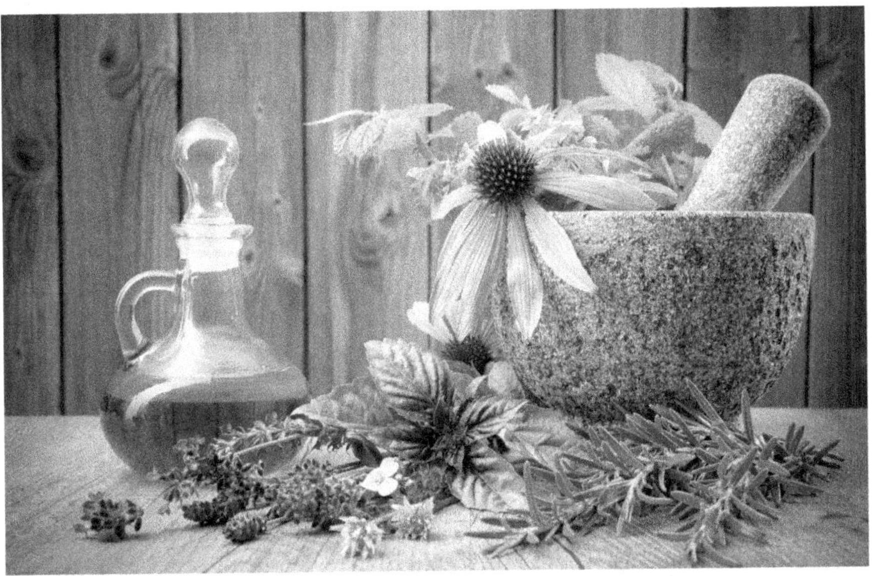

Introduction

In this chapter, we will delve into the deep waters of the beneficial properties of herbs, examining in detail how these extraordinary plants can significantly contribute to our well-being in various aspects of daily life.

Powerful Antioxidants for Overall Health

Numerous herbs, rich in antioxidants, play a fundamental role in promoting overall health. From green tea, known for its antioxidant catechins, to rosemary, offering anti-aging benefits, we will explore in depth how these properties can protect our cells from oxidative damage, contributing to healthy aging and robust well-being.

Calming Effects and Stress Reduction

Some herbs, including lavender, peppermint, and chamomile, are celebrated for their calming and stress-reducing properties. We will delve into how these plants can act on the nervous system, promote mental and physical relaxation, and tangibly contribute to the management of daily stress.

Digestive Support and Appetite Regulation

Herbs can play a significant role in supporting the digestive system and regulating appetite. We will examine how mint, licorice, and fennel can alleviate common digestive disturbances such as indigestion and bloating, contributing to a natural balance in appetite.

Enhancement of Concentration and Cognitive Functions

Certain herbs, such as bicep, ginkgo balboa, and sage, are associated with improving concentration and cognitive functions. We will explore how these plants can positively influence the brain, supporting memory and mental clarity.

Antibacterial and Antiviral Properties

Several herbs, like garlic, eucalyptus, and oregano, possess antibacterial and antiviral properties. We will examine how these plants can be proactively used to strengthen the immune system and prevent infections, offering a natural defence against common pathogens.

Alleviating Respiratory Issues with Expectorant Herbs

Herbs like ivy, licorice root, and thyme can play a crucial role in soothing respiratory issues such as coughs and colds. We will explore how these plants can contribute to clearing the airways, improving breathing, and promoting lung well-being.

Supporting Skin Health with Dermo protective Herbs

Herbs like calendula, aloe Vera, and lavender are widely used to support skin health. We will analyze how these plants can moisturize, soothe, and protect the skin from irritations and skin conditions, providing a solid foundation for skin well-being.

Sleep Regulation with Relaxing Herbs

Beyond improving sleep quality, some herbs, including valerian, passionflower, and lemon balm, can be used to regulate sleep patterns. We will examine how these plants can promote regular and restorative sleep, contributing to a more balanced sleep routine.

Conclusion

This chapter has shed light on the diverse beneficial properties of herbs, demonstrating how nature provides a vast arsenal of resources to enhance our health and well-being. In the next chapter, we will explore how to practically integrate these properties into our daily lives for a holistic approach to wellness.

CHAPTER 4

Phytotherapy

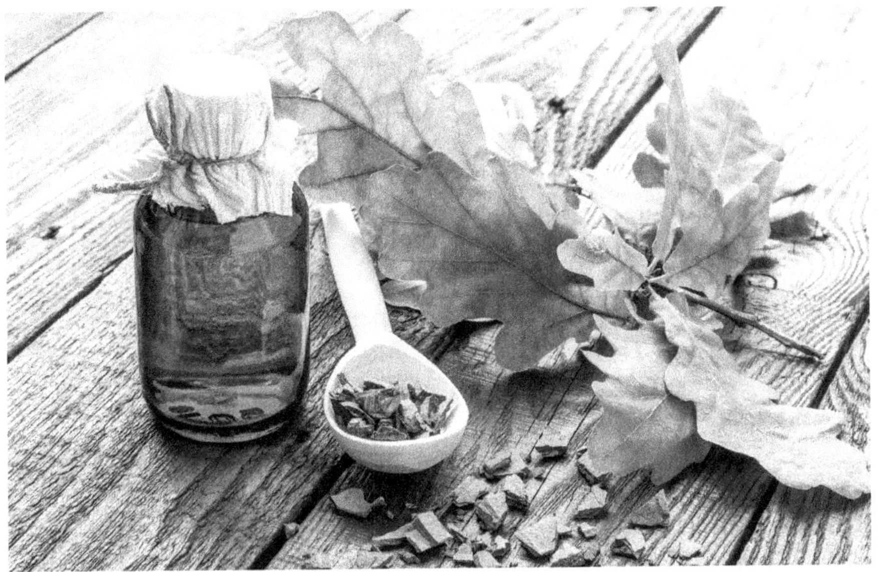

Phytotherapy is a discipline that utilizes plant extracts, such as herbs and plants, to prevent, alleviate, or treat health disorders. This approach is based on tradition and the use of natural compounds found in plants to promote well-being. Medicinal herbs are selected for their beneficial properties and are used in various forms, including herbal teas, tinctures, capsules, or extracts.

It's important to emphasize that phytotherapy should be practiced with care, taking into account individual characteristics and consulting a healthcare professional, especially if taking medications or having pre-existing health conditions. Phytotherapy can be part of a holistic approach to health, contributing to overall well-being through the mindful use of medicinal plants.

1. **Adaptogenic Herbs:** These herbs help the body adapt to stress and promote overall balance.
2. **Detoxifying Herbs:** Herbs that support the body's natural detoxification processes, aiding in the elimination of toxins.

3. **Digestive Herbs:** Plants that promote healthy digestion and support gastrointestinal functions.
4. **Immune-Boosting Herbs:** Herbs known for enhancing the immune system and promoting resistance to infections.
5. **Nervine Herbs:** Herbs that have a calming or tonifying effect on the nervous system, helping to manage stress.
6. **Anti-Inflammatory Herbs:** Plants with anti-inflammatory properties that can help alleviate inflammation in the body.
7. **Antioxidant-Rich Herbs:** Herbs that are rich in antioxidants, supporting the body in combating oxidative stress.
8. **Hormonal-Balancing Herbs:** Herbs that may help regulate hormonal imbalances and support endocrine health.
9. **Diuretic Herbs:** Herbs that promote urine production, supporting kidney function and fluid balance.
10. **Circulatory Herbs:** Plants that support healthy blood circulation and cardiovascular function.

Phytotherapy for the Respiratory System

In the field of herbal medicine, phytotherapy emerges as a potent ally in addressing various respiratory issues. From common colds and persistent coughs to conditions like asthma and sinusitis, herbal remedies offer a holistic approach to respiratory health. Plants with expectorant properties, such as thyme and licorice root, aid in relieving congestion and facilitating easier breathing. Additionally, anti-inflammatory herbs like turmeric and ginger contribute to reducing irritation in the respiratory tract. Herbs like eucalyptus and peppermint, renowned for their soothing qualities, can bring relief to symptoms associated with asthma and sinusitis. This chapter will explore the diverse herbal options available for promoting respiratory well-being and managing a range of respiratory disorders.

Phytotherapy for the Digestive System

In the realm of herbal medicine, phytotherapy emerges as a valuable resource for addressing digestive system disorders. From common indigestion and bloating to more complex gastrointestinal issues, herbal remedies offer a natural approach to promote digestive health.

Herbs like peppermint and fennel, with their carminative properties, help alleviate discomfort caused by gas and abdominal bloating. Plants like chamomile and licorice, with their anti-inflammatory and soothing properties, can contribute to reducing inflammation and soothing the gastrointestinal tract. This chapter will explore a variety of herbs with potential benefits for the digestive system, providing natural solutions to enhance digestion and address common issues related to the gastrointestinal tract.

Phytotherapy for the Cardiovascular

Phytotherapy emerges as a valuable resource in supporting cardiovascular health, providing a natural approach to maintaining the well-being of the heart and blood vessels. Herbs such as garlic, with its hypotensive properties, can contribute to regulating blood pressure. Hawthorn is known for its calming effect on the heart and can be used to support cardiac health. Omega-3s found in fish oil are often integrated into phytotherapy to promote cardiovascular system health. This chapter will explore a variety of herbs and natural remedies used in phytotherapy to enhance heart and blood vessel health, offering a holistic approach to cardiovascular health management.

Phytotherapy for the Nervous System

Phytotherapy emerges as a relevant resource in promoting the well-being of the nervous system, offering a natural approach to support mental and neural health. Herbs such as valerian and passionflower are known for their calming and relaxing properties, aiding in stress management and promoting sleep. Bacopa and ginkgo biloba are used to enhance cognitive function and support memory. Plants like lavender and chamomile can soothe nerves and reduce anxiety. This chapter will explore a range of herbs and natural remedies used in phytotherapy to promote the balance of the nervous system, providing a holistic approach to maintaining mental health and neural support.

Phytotherapy for the Urinary System

Phytotherapy, or the use of medicinal plants, offers natural solutions to promote the health and balance of the urinary system. Various herbs are known for their diuretic, anti-inflammatory, and antimicrobial properties, contributing to the well-being of the kidneys and urinary tract. Popular herbs in urinary phytotherapy include nettle, parsley, cranberry, and dandelion, each offering specific benefits for urinary health. It's essential to approach phytotherapy with care, considering individual health conditions and consulting a healthcare professional for personalized guidance.

CHAPTER 5

Herbs

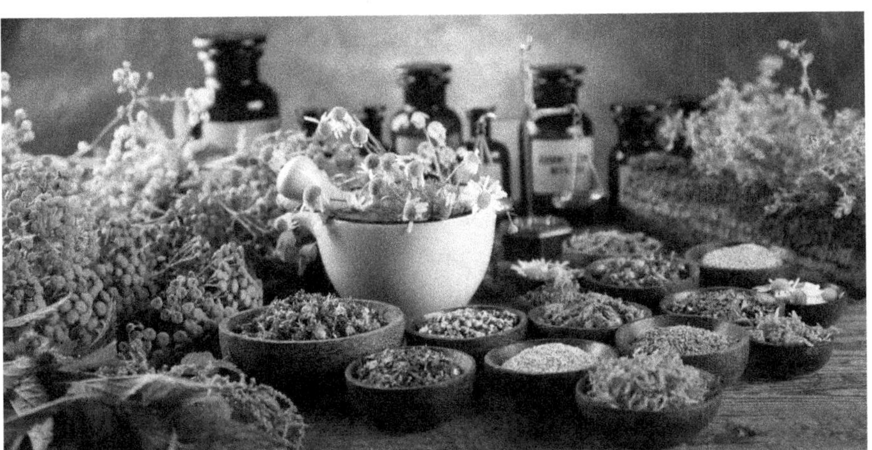

Tarragon

Tarragon, also known as Dragoncello, is a culinary herb with a distinctive flavor that is often used in French cuisine. There are two main types of tarragon: Russian tarragon (Artemisia dracunculoides) and French tarragon (Artemisia dracunculus var. sativa). French tarragon is the more widely used and preferred variety for culinary purposes due to its superior flavor.

Here are some key points about tarragon:

1. **Flavor Profile:** Tarragon has a unique flavor that is often described as a combination of anise and licorice. It adds a subtle, sweet, and slightly peppery taste to dishes.
2. **Culinary Uses:** Tarragon is a popular herb in French cuisine, where it is a key ingredient in the classic fines herbes blend. It pairs well with poultry, fish, eggs, and vegetables. It is often used to flavor sauces, dressings, and vinegar.
3. **Growing Conditions:** Tarragon prefers well-drained soil and plenty of sunlight. It can be grown in gardens or in containers.

French tarragon is typically propagated through cuttings, as it rarely produces viable seeds.

4. **Harvesting:** The leaves of tarragon can be harvested as needed, and the flavor is most intense just before the plant flowers. Harvesting the leaves regularly can encourage bushier growth.

5. **Preserving Tarragon:** Tarragon can be preserved by drying or freezing. While drying retains more of the flavor, freezing can be a convenient way to preserve the herb without losing too much of its taste.

6. **Health Benefits:** Tarragon is believed to have some health benefits. It contains certain compounds that may have anti-inflammatory and antioxidant properties. Additionally, it has been used in traditional medicine for its digestive and appetite-stimulating properties.

7. **Medicinal Uses:** In traditional medicine, tarragon has been used for various purposes, including as a remedy for digestive issues and as a mild sedative. However, its medicinal uses are not as well-established or widely recognized as its culinary uses.

When using tarragon in cooking, it's best to add it towards the end of the cooking process to preserve its delicate flavor. Whether fresh or dried, tarragon can be a delightful addition to a variety of dishes, imparting a distinct and aromatic taste.

Alfalfa

Alfalfa (Medicago sativa) is a flowering plant that belongs to the legume family (Fabaceae). It is known for its small, clover-like leaves and is commonly used as a forage crop for livestock. However, alfalfa also has various uses and benefits for human consumption. Here are some key points about alfalfa:

1. **Forage Crop:** Alfalfa is primarily cultivated as a forage crop for livestock, including cattle, horses, and poultry. Its high nutritional content makes it a valuable feed, providing proteins, vitamins, and minerals for animals.

2. **Nutrient Content:** Alfalfa is rich in nutrients, including vitamins A, C, E, and K, as well as various B vitamins. It also contains essential minerals such as calcium, magnesium, phosphorus, and

iron. The plant's nutritional profile makes it a popular choice for inclusion in animal feeds and as a supplement for humans.

3. **Sprouts:** Alfalfa sprouts are a common and popular addition to salads and sandwiches. These sprouts are produced by germinating alfalfa seeds and are known for their mild, nutty flavor. They are a good source of vitamins, minerals, and antioxidants.

4. **Health Benefits:** Alfalfa has been traditionally used in herbal medicine for its potential health benefits. It is believed to have diuretic properties and may be used to support kidney health. Additionally, some people use alfalfa supplements for conditions such as arthritis and high cholesterol, although more research is needed to confirm these potential benefits.

5. **Drought-Tolerant Crop:** Alfalfa is known for its ability to withstand drought conditions better than many other crops. Its deep root system allows it to access water from lower soil layers, making it a resilient forage option in areas with limited water availability.

6. **Cover Crop:** In agriculture, alfalfa is sometimes used as a cover crop to improve soil fertility. Its deep roots can help break up compacted soil, and its ability to fix nitrogen from the air can enhance soil fertility.

7. **Hay Production:** Alfalfa is commonly grown for hay production, providing a high-quality forage material for livestock. It is cut and dried before being baled for storage and later use as animal feed.

8. **Herbal Tea:** Alfalfa leaves are used to make herbal tea. The tea is mild in flavor and is sometimes consumed for its potential health benefits, including as a source of vitamins and minerals.

While alfalfa has many positive aspects, it's worth noting that some people may be allergic to alfalfa or its seeds. As with any herbal supplement, it's advisable to consult with a healthcare professional before using alfalfa for medicinal purposes, especially if you have existing health conditions or are taking other medications.

Lemon Balm

Lemon balm (Melissa officinalis) is a fragrant herb from the mint family (Lamiaceae). It is known for its lemony aroma and is widely used for culinary, medicinal, and ornamental purposes. Here are some key points about lemon balm:

1. **Aroma and Flavor:** Lemon balm has a distinct lemon fragrance, which is released when the leaves are crushed. The flavor is mildly citrusy, making it a popular choice for culinary applications.
2. **Culinary Uses:** Lemon balm is often used in cooking and baking. It can be used to flavor salads, soups, sauces, desserts, and beverages. It pairs well with fish, poultry, and vegetables. Additionally, it is used to make herbal teas and infusions.
3. **Medicinal Uses:** Lemon balm has been traditionally used in herbal medicine for various purposes. It is believed to have calming and relaxing properties and is often used to help alleviate stress, anxiety, and insomnia. It may also be used for digestive issues and as a mild antiviral.
4. **Herbal Tea:** Lemon balm is commonly used to make a soothing and aromatic herbal tea. The tea is often consumed to promote relaxation and relieve stress. It can be enjoyed on its own or blended with other herbs.
5. **Anti-Anxiety Effects:** Some studies suggest that lemon balm may have mild anti-anxiety effects. The herb is thought to interact with receptors in the brain associated with relaxation and mood regulation.
6. **Growing Conditions:** Lemon balm is a hardy and easy-to-grow herb. It prefers well-drained soil and partial to full sunlight. It can be grown in gardens or in containers.
7. **Propagation:** Lemon balm can be propagated through seeds, cuttings, or division of established plants. It has a tendency to spread, so it's advisable to plant it in a controlled area or in containers.
8. **Companion Plant:** In gardening, lemon balm is sometimes used as a companion plant. It is believed to attract beneficial insects and repel certain pests.
9. **Cosmetic and Aromatic Uses:** Lemon balm extracts or oils are sometimes used in cosmetics and aromatherapy due to their pleasant scent. They may be found in products such as perfumes, lotions, and essential oils.
10. **Caution:** While lemon balm is generally considered safe, individuals with thyroid conditions should use it cautiously as it may have a mild effect on thyroid function. As with any herbal remedy,

it's advisable to consult with a healthcare professional, especially if you are pregnant, nursing, or taking medications.

Lemon balm is a versatile herb that adds a refreshing and citrusy touch to both culinary and herbal preparations. It's valued not only for its flavor but also for its potential calming effects.

Fennel

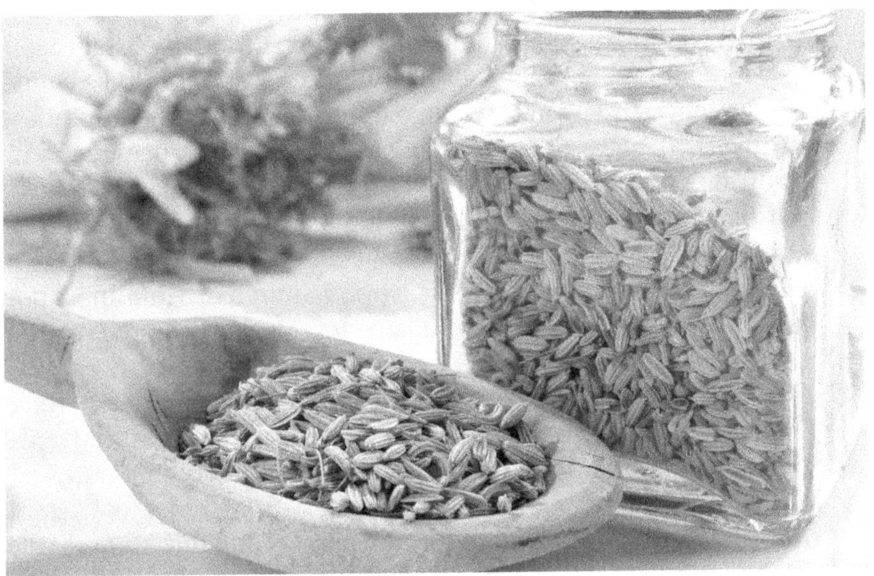

Fennel (Foeniculum vulgare) is a flowering plant in the carrot family (Apiaceae) that is widely used for its aromatic leaves, seeds, and bulb. It has a sweet and licorice-like flavor and is employed in various culinary and medicinal applications. Here are some key points about fennel:

1. **Bulb:** The fennel bulb is a crunchy, white or pale green vegetable with a mild anise or licorice flavor. It can be sliced and used raw in salads or cooked in a variety of dishes such as soups, stews, and stir-fries.
2. **Leaves (Foliage):** Fennel leaves, also known as fronds, are feathery and delicate. They can be used as an herb to add flavor to salads, soups, and dishes with fish or poultry.
3. **Seeds:** Fennel seeds are small, oval-shaped, and brown. They have

a strong anise flavor and are commonly used as a spice in cooking and baking. Fennel seeds are also popular for making herbal teas.

4. **Culinary Uses:** Fennel is a versatile ingredient used in both savory and sweet dishes. It complements the flavors of fish, pork, chicken, and various vegetables. It can be roasted, grilled, sautéed, or eaten raw, depending on the culinary application.

5. **Herbal Tea:** Fennel tea is made by infusing fennel seeds in hot water. It is known for its mild, aromatic flavor and is sometimes consumed for its potential digestive benefits. Fennel tea is caffeine-free and can be enjoyed hot or cold.

6. **Digestive Benefits:** Fennel has been traditionally used to aid digestion. It may help alleviate bloating, indigestion, and gas. Some people chew fennel seeds after meals for their digestive properties.

7. **Medicinal Uses:** Beyond digestion, fennel has been used in traditional medicine for various purposes. It is believed to have antioxidant properties and may have mild anti-inflammatory effects.

8. **Nutrient Content:** Fennel is a good source of vitamin C, potassium, and dietary fiber. It is also low in calories, making it a healthy addition to a balanced diet.

9. **Growing Conditions:** Fennel is a hardy herb that prefers well-drained soil and full sunlight. It can be grown from seeds or transplants and is suitable for both garden beds and containers.

10. **Culinary Pairings:** Fennel pairs well with ingredients like citrus, olives, tomatoes, and herbs like parsley and dill. Its versatile flavor makes it a valuable addition to a wide range of recipes.

11. **Wild Fennel:** In some regions, wild fennel (Foeniculum vulgare var. dulce) grows abundantly. The plant is often considered an invasive species but is also harvested for culinary and medicinal purposes.

Fennel is appreciated not only for its culinary versatility but also for its potential health benefits. It adds a unique and aromatic dimension to dishes and is a valuable ingredient in many cuisines around the world.

Summer Savory

Summer savory (Satureja hortensis) is a herb that belongs to the mint family (Lamiaceae). It is known for its aromatic leaves and is commonly used as a culinary herb, adding a warm and peppery flavor to various dishes. Here are some key points about summer savory:

1. **Flavor Profile:** Summer savory has a mild and peppery taste with a hint of thyme and mint. It is less pungent than its relative, winter savory, making it a popular choice for culinary use.

2. **Culinary Uses:** Summer savory is a versatile herb used to flavor a variety of dishes. It complements the flavors of beans, vegetables, meats, and poultry. It is often included in spice blends like herbes de Provence and fines herbes. Additionally, it can be used in salads, soups, stews, and stuffing.

3. **Drying and Preserving:** Summer savory retains its flavor well when dried, and dried leaves can be crumbled and used in cooking. It is also possible to freeze the herb to preserve its flavor.

4. **Growing Conditions:** Summer savory is an annual herb that is relatively easy to grow. It prefers well-drained soil and full sunlight. It can be grown in gardens or containers.

5. **Propagation:** Summer savory can be grown from seeds, and it typically germinates quickly. It is also possible to propagate the herb through cuttings.

6. **Harvesting:** The leaves of summer savory can be harvested as needed once the plant has reached a sufficient size. Harvesting the leaves just before the plant flowers can help preserve the best flavor.

7. **Medicinal Uses:** While summer savory is primarily used as a culinary herb, it has been traditionally used in herbal medicine for its potential digestive and antimicrobial properties. However, its medicinal uses are not as well-documented or widely recognized as its culinary uses.

8. **Companion Planting:** Summer savory is sometimes used in companion planting to deter certain pests. It is believed to repel bean beetles and other insects that can affect legumes.

9. **Similarity to Winter Savory:** Summer savory is related to winter savory (Satureja montana), but the two herbs have different flavor profiles. Winter savory tends to have a stronger, more resinous taste and is often used in meat dishes and stews.

10. **Traditional Use:** Summer savory has a long history of use in traditional cuisines, particularly in Mediterranean and European dishes. It is a common herb in French, Italian, and Greek cooking.

Whether used fresh or dried, summer savory adds a delightful and aromatic flavor to a variety of dishes. It's a popular choice for herb gardens and is appreciated for its ability to enhance the taste of many culinary creations.

Lavender

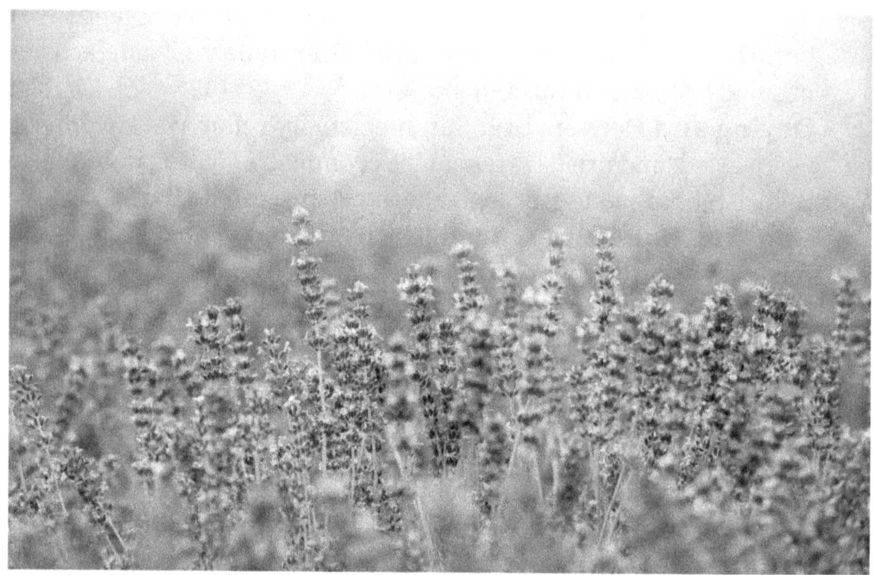

Lavender (Lavandula) is a well-known aromatic herb that belongs to the mint family (Lamiaceae). It is prized for its fragrant flowers, which are commonly used in a variety of applications, including culinary, medicinal, and cosmetic. Here are some key points about lavender:

1. **Aroma:** Lavender is renowned for its sweet, floral, and herbaceous aroma. The essential oil extracted from lavender flowers is widely used in perfumes, aromatherapy, and various cosmetic products.
2. **Culinary Uses:** Culinary lavender is used to flavor both sweet and savory dishes. Lavender-infused honey, teas, and desserts, such as lavender-flavored ice cream and cookies, are popular culinary applications. It's important to use culinary-grade lavender to ensure it is free of pesticides and safe for consumption.
3. **Varieties:** There are several species and cultivars of lavender,

each with its unique characteristics. English lavender (Lavandula angustifolia) is often preferred for culinary purposes due to its milder flavor.

4. **Medicinal Uses:** Lavender has a long history of use in traditional medicine. It is believed to have calming and relaxing properties and may be used to alleviate stress, anxiety, and insomnia. Lavender oil is also applied topically for its potential antiseptic and anti-inflammatory properties.

5. **Aromatherapy:** Lavender essential oil is a popular choice for aromatherapy. Inhaling the scent of lavender is thought to have calming effects and may help promote relaxation and improve sleep.

6. **Cosmetic and Personal Care Products:** Lavender is a common ingredient in a wide range of cosmetic and personal care products, including soaps, lotions, shampoos, and bath oils. Its soothing properties make it a popular choice for skincare.

7. **Growing Conditions:** Lavender plants thrive in well-drained soil and full sunlight. They are known for their drought resistance and are often cultivated in gardens, landscapes, and containers.

8. **Harvesting:** Lavender flowers are typically harvested when they are in full bloom. The timing of the harvest can affect the flavor and fragrance of the lavender.

9. **Drying Lavender:** To preserve lavender for later use, the flowers can be dried. Hanging bunches of lavender upside down in a dry, dark place is a common method of drying.

10. **Lavender in Crafts:** Dried lavender is often used in crafts and DIY projects, such as sachets, potpourri, and homemade candles. The aromatic properties of dried lavender make it a popular choice for adding a pleasant scent to various items.

11. **Lavender as a Landscape Plant:** Lavender is often planted in gardens and landscapes for its ornamental value. The plants are known for their fragrant flowers, silvery foliage, and the ability to attract pollinators.

It's important to note that while lavender is generally considered safe, some individuals may be allergic to it. Additionally, pregnant or nursing women should exercise caution with the use of lavender essential oil. As with any herbal remedy, it's advisable to consult with a healthcare professional, especially if you have existing health.

Maca

Maca (Lepidium meyenii), sometimes referred to as Peruvian ginseng, is a plant native to the Andes mountains in Peru. It has been cultivated and consumed as a food source for centuries in the Andean region, particularly in Peru. The root of the maca plant is the part that is primarily used for its potential health benefits. Here are some key points about maca:

1. **Nutritional Content:** Maca is rich in various nutrients, including carbohydrates, fiber, protein, vitamins (such as B vitamins), and minerals (such as iron, potassium, and calcium).

2. **Adaptogen:** Maca is often classified as an adaptogen, a term used for substances that may help the body adapt to stressors. It is believed to have the potential to support the body's response to physical and mental stress.

3. **Traditional Use:** In traditional Peruvian medicine, maca has been used for a variety of purposes, including enhancing stamina, energy, and fertility. It is also believed to have aphrodisiac properties.

4. **Hormone Regulation:** Some studies suggest that maca may have a balancing effect on hormones, particularly in relation to reproductive hormones such as estrogen, progesterone, and testosterone. It's important to note that research in this area is still ongoing, and more evidence is needed.

5. **Libido and Sexual Function:** Maca is often promoted as a natural remedy to support libido and sexual function. Some individuals take maca supplements for these purposes, but the scientific evidence supporting its effectiveness is limited.

6. **Energy and Endurance:** Traditional uses of maca also include its role in increasing energy and stamina. Athletes and individuals engaged in physical activities sometimes use maca as a natural supplement to support endurance.

7. **Forms of Consumption:** Maca is available in various forms, including powder, capsules, and extracts. The powdered form is a common choice, and it can be added to smoothies, beverages, or food.

8. **Colors of Maca:** Maca roots come in different colors, including yellow, red, and black. Each color is believed to have slightly different properties, with yellow maca being more common and

the other colors considered more rare and sometimes associated with specific benefits.

9. **Caution and Considerations:** While maca is generally considered safe for most people when consumed in moderate amounts as a food, there is limited research on its long-term safety, especially in supplement form. As with any supplement, it's advisable to consult with a healthcare professional before adding maca or any new dietary supplement to your routine, especially if you have pre-existing health conditions or are taking medications.

10. **Culinary Uses:** In addition to its potential health benefits, maca is also used as a food ingredient in Peru. It has a nutty and earthy flavor and is sometimes added to soups, stews, and various dishes.

It's crucial to approach the use of maca or any other dietary supplement with caution, understanding that individual responses can vary. If considering maca for specific health goals, consulting with a healthcare professional is recommended to ensure its appropriateness for your situation.

Yerba Maté

Yerba mate (Ilex paraguariensis) is a plant native to South America, particularly in Argentina, Paraguay, Uruguay, and southern Brazil. The leaves of the yerba mate plant are used to make a beverage known as mate. Here are some key points about yerba mate:

1. **Preparation:** The traditional method of preparing yerba mate involves placing dried leaves and twigs in a hollowed-out gourd (mate) and adding hot (but not boiling) water. The drink is then sipped through a metal straw called a bombilla.

2. **Caffeine Content:** Yerba mate contains caffeine, theobromine, and other stimulants, making it a popular choice for those seeking a natural energy boost. However, the caffeine content is typically lower than that of coffee.

3. **Flavor Profile:** Yerba mate has a distinctive, earthy, and somewhat bitter flavor. It can be an acquired taste for some, and its flavor can vary depending on factors such as the type of leaves, region of cultivation, and the method of processing.

4. **Nutritional Content:** Yerba mate is rich in antioxidants, vitamins

(such as vitamins A, B1, B2, B3, B5, B6, C, and E), and minerals (including calcium, iron, magnesium, manganese, phosphorus, potassium, and zinc). It also contains polyphenols, which contribute to its antioxidant properties.

5. **Cultural Significance:** Yerba mate holds cultural significance in South America, particularly in Argentina, where it is a common social beverage. Sharing mate is a communal practice, and it is often enjoyed in social settings among friends and family.

6. **Health Benefits:** Yerba mate has been associated with various health benefits, including improved mental alertness, enhanced focus, and increased energy. It also contains compounds with potential anti-inflammatory and antioxidant properties. Some studies suggest that yerba mate may have cardiovascular benefits and could aid in weight management.

7. **Social Ritual:** Drinking yerba mate is often considered a social ritual. The mate is passed around, with each person taking turns sipping from the shared gourd. This communal practice is deeply rooted in South American culture.

8. **Commercial Products:** Yerba mate is not only consumed in its traditional form but is also used as an ingredient in various commercial products, including energy drinks, teas, and dietary supplements.

9. **Terminology:** The term "mate" can refer to both the beverage and the hollowed-out gourd used for drinking it. The plant itself is called yerba mate, with "yerba" meaning herb or plant.

10. **Mate in Different Forms:** While the traditional preparation involves loose leaves in a gourd, yerba mate is also available in tea bags and ready-to-drink formats, making it more convenient for those who may not be familiar with the traditional preparation method.

11. **Cautions:** While yerba mate is generally considered safe for most people, excessive consumption may have potential health risks, similar to those associated with caffeine intake. It's advisable to moderate yerba mate consumption, especially for individuals sensitive to caffeine or those with certain health conditions.

As with any herbal beverage, individual responses to yerba mate can vary. If you have concerns about its impact on your health or if you have pre-existing health conditions, it's recommended to consult with a healthcare professional before incorporating yerba mate into your regular routine.

Bobinsana

Bobinsana, scientifically known as Calliandra angustifolia, is a plant native to the Amazon rainforest in South America. It has been traditionally used by indigenous peoples for its medicinal properties. Here are some key points about bobinsana:

1. **Traditional Use:** Indigenous communities in the Amazon rainforest, particularly in Peru, Colombia, and Ecuador, have used bobinsana for various traditional purposes. It is often prepared as an herbal infusion or tincture.
2. **Medicinal Uses:** Bobinsana is believed to have a range of medicinal properties. It is traditionally used to address conditions such as arthritis, rheumatism, respiratory issues, and menstrual disorders. Additionally, it is sometimes used for its potential psychoactive and energetic effects.
3. **Psychoactive Properties:** In traditional Amazonian medicine, bobinsana is sometimes considered a plant teacher or a plant ally with spirit-enhancing properties. It is believed to have subtle psychoactive effects that may induce altered states of consciousness during ceremonial use.
4. **Energetic and Spiritual Uses:** Bobinsana is often used in traditional healing ceremonies for its purported energetic and spiritual properties. It is sometimes considered a plant teacher that can aid in spiritual development, introspection, and connecting with the natural world.
5. **Preparation:** The most common way to consume bobinsana is by making a decoction or infusion from the leaves and stem bark. The liquid is often ingested orally during traditional ceremonies. Additionally, bobinsana may be used in combination with other plants for specific healing purposes.
6. **Appearance:** The bobinsana plant is a shrub or small tree with compound leaves and pink to reddish flowers. It is a member of the legume family (Fabaceae).
7. **Conservation Concerns:** Due to increasing interest in traditional Amazonian plant medicines, there are concerns about

overharvesting and unsustainable harvesting practices of plants like bobinsana. Sustainable and ethical harvesting practices are important to ensure the conservation of these valuable plant species.

8. **Cultural Importance:** Plants like bobinsana play a significant role in the cultural practices and beliefs of indigenous communities in the Amazon. Traditional healers, known as shamans or curanderos, often work with plant medicines in their healing practices.

9. **Research and Studies:** While there is a long history of traditional use, scientific research on bobinsana is limited. The plant has not been extensively studied in terms of its pharmacological properties, and more research is needed to understand its potential benefits and risks.

10. **Caution:** As with any traditional plant medicine, caution is advised, especially if considering the use of bobinsana outside of its traditional context. It's crucial to approach the use of such plants with respect and under the guidance of knowledgeable individuals, such as traditional healers or herbalists.

It's important to note that the information provided here is based on traditional knowledge and practices. If you are considering the use of bobinsana or any other plant for medicinal purposes, it's recommended to consult with qualified healthcare professionals or experienced practitioners who are knowledgeable about traditional plant medicine.

Thai Kratom

Kratom (Mitragyna speciosa) is a tropical tree native to Southeast Asia, including Thailand, Malaysia, Indonesia, and Papua New Guinea. The leaves of the kratom tree have been traditionally used for various medicinal and recreational purposes. Thai kratom specifically refers to kratom that originates from Thailand.

Here are some key points about Thai kratom:

1. **Varieties:** Thai kratom is often categorized based on the color of the veins in its leaves, which can be red, green, or white. Each variety is associated with slightly different effects, and individual responses can vary.

> » **Red Thai Kratom:** Generally associated with relaxation and pain relief.
> » **Green Thai Kratom:** Often reported to provide a balance between energy and relaxation.
> » **White Thai Kratom:** Typically associated with increased energy and focus.

2. **Alkaloids:** Kratom leaves contain various alkaloids, including mitragynine and 7-hydroxymitragynine, which are believed to be responsible for the plant's effects. The concentrations of these alkaloids can vary among different kratom strains.

3. **Traditional Use:** Kratom has a long history of traditional use in Southeast Asia. It has been used by indigenous communities for its stimulant and pain-relieving properties. In Thailand, kratom has been traditionally chewed or brewed into a tea.

4. **Effects:** The effects of Thai kratom, like other kratom strains, can vary depending on the dose and individual sensitivity. Low doses may be associated with increased alertness and sociability, while higher doses may lead to sedation and pain relief.

5. **Stimulant and Analgesic Properties:** Kratom is known for its dual nature, acting as a stimulant at lower doses and as an analgesic (pain reliever) at higher doses. Users often describe increased focus, mood enhancement, and mild euphoria at lower doses.

6. **Availability:** Kratom, including Thai kratom, is available in various forms, including powdered leaves, capsules, and extracts. It is also sold under different brand names.

7. **Legality:** The legal status of kratom varies by country and jurisdiction. While it is legal in some places, there are areas where it is banned or restricted. Regulations may change, so it's essential to be aware of the legal status of kratom in your location.

8. **Controversy and Health Concerns:** Kratom has been a subject of controversy and has raised health concerns, including the potential for dependence and addiction. Additionally, there have been reports of adverse effects, including nausea, vomiting, and other side effects. Long-term health effects and safety have not been thoroughly studied.

9. **Caution and Responsible Use:** Due to the lack of regulation and research, caution is advised when using kratom. It's essential to start with low doses, be aware of individual tolerance, and avoid

excessive or frequent use. Individuals with pre-existing health conditions or those taking medications should consult with a healthcare professional before using kratom.

10. **Cultural Context:** While kratom has cultural and historical significance in Southeast Asia, its use outside of its traditional cultural context has led to debates about its safety and regulation in various parts of the world.

As with any substance, it's important to approach the use of Thai kratom responsibly and be aware of potential risks. If considering the use of kratom, it's advisable to educate oneself, seek information from reliable sources, and, if necessary, consult with healthcare professionals.

Guarana

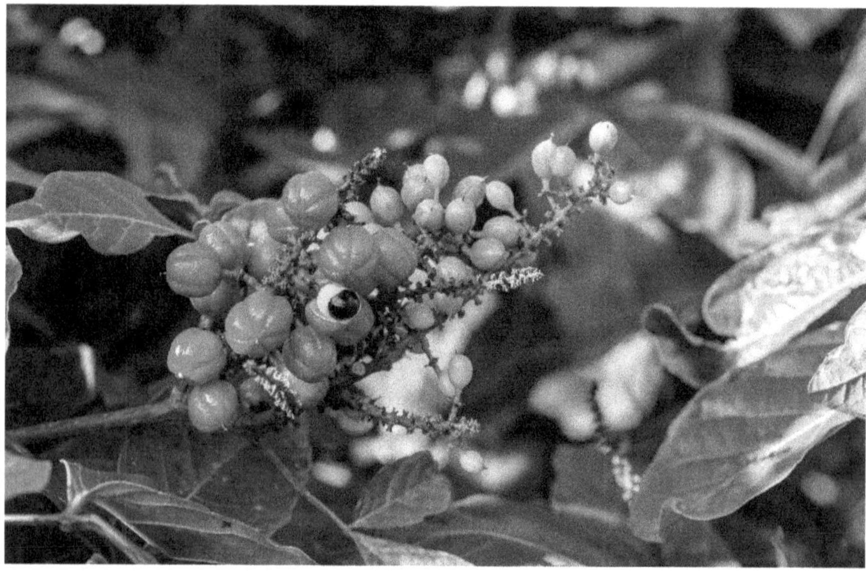

Guarana (Paullinia cupana) is a climbing plant native to the Amazon basin in Brazil. It is best known for its seeds, which contain caffeine and other natural compounds. Guarana has a long history of traditional use among indigenous tribes in the Amazon rainforest, and it has gained popularity worldwide for its stimulant properties and potential health benefits. Here are some key points about guarana:

1. **Caffeine Content:** Guarana seeds are rich in caffeine, and they contain higher concentrations of caffeine compared to coffee beans. The caffeine in guarana is often released more slowly in the body, providing a more sustained and prolonged energy boost.

2. **Traditional Use:** Indigenous people in the Amazon have used guarana for centuries as a natural stimulant. It has been traditionally consumed in the form of a paste or beverage made from crushed guarana seeds. The plant has cultural and ritual significance in some Amazonian tribes.

3. **Stimulant Properties:** The caffeine content in guarana is the primary reason for its stimulant properties. It is known to enhance alertness, reduce fatigue, and improve cognitive function. Some people use guarana as a natural alternative to coffee or energy drinks.

4. **Energizing Supplements:** Guarana is commonly used as an ingredient in energy drinks, dietary supplements, and herbal formulations aimed at boosting energy and mental alertness. It is often included in combination with other herbs, vitamins, and minerals.

5. **Antioxidant Properties:** In addition to caffeine, guarana contains other natural compounds, including tannins and catechins, which have antioxidant properties. Antioxidants help neutralize free radicals in the body and may contribute to overall health.

6. **Weight Loss and Metabolism:** Guarana has been marketed as a supplement for weight loss due to its stimulant effects on metabolism. Some studies suggest that caffeine can increase thermogenesis (the body's production of heat), which may contribute to weight loss.

7. **Mood Enhancement:** Caffeine, as found in guarana, is known to have mood-enhancing effects. It can increase the release of certain neurotransmitters, such as dopamine and serotonin, which play a role in mood regulation.

8. **Formulations and Dosage:** Guarana is available in various forms, including capsules, tablets, extracts, and energy drinks. The appropriate dosage can vary based on the formulation and individual tolerance. It's important to follow recommended guidelines and avoid excessive intake.

9. **Caution:** While guarana is generally considered safe when consumed in moderation, excessive caffeine intake can lead to side

effects such as insomnia, nervousness, and increased heart rate. Individuals with certain health conditions, such as cardiovascular issues, should exercise caution and consult with a healthcare professional before using guarana supplements.

10. **Regulatory Status:** The regulatory status of guarana supplements varies by country. In some regions, it is considered a dietary supplement, while in others, it may be subject to specific regulations.

As with any herbal supplement, it's important to approach guarana with caution, particularly if considering it as part of a routine or for specific health goals. Consulting with a healthcare professional is advisable, especially for individuals with pre-existing health conditions or those taking medications.

Cola Nut

Cola nut refers to the seeds of the cola tree (Cola spp.), particularly those of two species: Cola acuminata and Cola nitida. These trees are native to the rainforests of West Africa. The seeds are known for their stimulating properties and are used as a source of caffeine. Here are some key points about cola nut:

1. **Caffeine Content:** Cola nuts are rich in caffeine, and they have been historically used as a natural stimulant. The caffeine content in cola nuts is similar to that in coffee beans.

2. **Traditional Use:** Cola nut has a long history of traditional use in West African cultures. It has been used in rituals, ceremonies, and social gatherings. Chewing or making infusions from cola nuts is a traditional practice to enjoy their stimulating effects.

3. **Culinary Use:** Cola nuts have been used as a flavoring agent in some traditional recipes and beverages. The flavor of the nuts is bitter and slightly astringent.

4. **Cola Beverages:** The use of cola nuts as a flavoring agent is most commonly associated with the creation of cola beverages. In the late 19th and early 20th centuries, cola drinks were originally formulated using extracts from cola nuts, along with other ingredients like coca leaves.

5. **Commercial Cola Drinks:** While cola nuts were initially used in the formulation of cola beverages, most commercial cola drinks

today use synthetic flavorings. The caffeine in these drinks is often derived from other sources.

6. **Stimulant Properties:** The caffeine in cola nuts provides stimulant effects, helping to increase alertness, reduce fatigue, and improve concentration. This is why cola drinks, even those without actual cola nut extracts, are often associated with providing a "pick-me-up" due to their caffeine content.

7. **Chemical Composition:** Besides caffeine, cola nuts contain other compounds such as theobromine and tannins. Theobromine is a stimulant found in chocolate and tea, and tannins contribute to the bitter taste of the nuts.

8. **Health Considerations:** Cola nut consumption should be approached with moderation, especially for individuals sensitive to caffeine. Excessive caffeine intake can lead to side effects such as insomnia, increased heart rate, and nervousness. Individuals with certain health conditions, such as cardiovascular issues, should consult with a healthcare professional before consuming cola nut products.

9. **Cultural Significance:** Cola nuts hold cultural and social significance in certain African traditions. They are sometimes exchanged as gifts, and their use is associated with hospitality.

10. **Conservation and Sustainability:** The demand for cola nuts has led to concerns about sustainability and conservation. In some regions, efforts are made to promote sustainable harvesting practices to ensure the long-term viability of cola trees.

While cola nuts continue to be used in some traditional contexts, the widespread use of synthetic flavorings and alternative sources of caffeine has diminished their role in the production of commercial cola beverages. It's important to be aware of the caffeine content and potential health implications when consuming products containing cola nuts or their extracts. As with any dietary consideration, consulting with a healthcare professional is advisable, especially for individuals with specific health concerns.

Ginseng

Ginseng refers to a group of perennial plants belonging to the genus Panax. The term "ginseng" is commonly used to describe two primary species: Asian or Korean ginseng (Panax ginseng) and American ginseng (Panax quinquefolius). These plants have been used in traditional medicine for centuries and are known for their potential health benefits. Here are some key points about ginseng:

Common Types of Ginseng

1. **Asian Ginseng (Panax ginseng):**

    » Also known as Korean ginseng or red ginseng.
    » Traditionally used in East Asia, particularly in traditional Chinese medicine (TCM) and Korean traditional medicine.
    » Often steamed and dried to produce red ginseng.
    » Adaptogenic properties are emphasized, helping the body adapt to stress.

2. **American Ginseng (Panax quinquefolius):**

    » Native to North America.
    » Traditionally used by Native American tribes and later adopted in Western herbal medicine.
    » Generally considered milder than Asian ginseng.
    » May be used for adaptogenic purposes and to support general well-being.

3. **Siberian Ginseng (Eleutherococcus senticosus):**

    » While often referred to as "Siberian ginseng," it is not a true ginseng (Panax).
    » Used in traditional medicine in Russia and China.
    » Known for adaptogenic properties.

Key Points

1. **Adaptogenic Properties:**

    » Ginseng is often classified as an adaptogen, a substance believed to help the body adapt to stress and promote overall well-being.
    » Adaptogens are thought to have a balancing effect on the body's systems.

2. **Active Compounds:**

   » Ginsenosides are the primary active compounds in ginseng.
   » The concentration of ginsenosides may vary depending on factors such as the species, age of the plant, and processing methods.

3. **Traditional Uses:**

   » In traditional medicine, ginseng has been used for various purposes, including boosting energy, improving cognitive function, and enhancing physical endurance.
   » Both Asian and American ginseng have been used to support the immune system and as general tonics.

4. **Cognitive Function:**

   » Some studies suggest that ginseng may have cognitive-enhancing effects, potentially benefiting memory and mental alertness.

5. **Physical Performance:**

   » Athletes and individuals involved in physical activities have sometimes used ginseng to improve endurance and reduce fatigue.

6. **Stress and Fatigue:**

   » Ginseng is often taken to combat stress and fatigue, with users reporting increased energy and reduced feelings of tiredness.

7. **Caution and Considerations:**

   » Ginseng is generally considered safe for short-term use in recommended doses.
   » Long-term safety and potential interactions with medications should be discussed with a healthcare professional.
   » Individuals with certain health conditions, such as diabetes or high blood pressure, should exercise caution.

8. **Forms of Consumption:**

   » Ginseng is available in various forms, including fresh or dried roots, extracts, capsules, and teas.

» Asian ginseng is sometimes steamed and dried to produce red ginseng, which is believed to have different properties.

9. **Regulatory Status:**

   » Ginseng supplements are widely available and are considered dietary supplements in many regions.
   » Quality can vary among products, so it's advisable to choose reputable brands.

10. **Individual Responses:**

- The effects of ginseng can vary among individuals, and its impact may be influenced by factors such as age, health status, and the presence of underlying conditions.

While ginseng has a long history of traditional use and some promising research, individual responses can vary. It's important for individuals considering ginseng supplementation to consult with a healthcare professional, especially if they have pre-existing health conditions or are taking medications.

Ephedra

Ephedra refers to a genus of plants that contains species known for their high content of ephedrine alkaloids, which have stimulant and thermogenic effects. One of the most well-known species in this genus is Ephedra sinica, also known as Ma Huang. Ephedrine, a compound found in ephedra, has been used historically in traditional medicine for its stimulant properties. However, it has also been associated with potential health risks, leading to regulatory restrictions in various countries.

Here are some key points about ephedra:

Historical and Traditional Use

1. **Traditional Medicine:** Ephedra has been used in traditional Chinese medicine for thousands of years. It was traditionally used

to treat conditions such as asthma, respiratory issues, and as a
general stimulant.

Key Components and Mechanism of Action

1. **Ephedrine Alkaloids:** Ephedra contains ephedrine and related
   alkaloids, which act as sympathomimetic compounds. Ephedrine
   can stimulate the central nervous system, increase heart rate, and
   dilate bronchial tubes.
2. **Stimulant Effects:** Ephedrine is known for its stimulant properties, which can lead to increased alertness, energy, and metabolism.
   It has been used as a component in weight-loss and energy-boosting
   supplements.

Health Concerns and Regulatory Actions

1. **Adverse Effects:** The use of ephedra-containing supplements
   has been associated with adverse effects such as increased heart
   rate, elevated blood pressure, insomnia, and gastrointestinal disturbances.
2. **Safety Concerns:** Serious health concerns, including cardiovascular events and deaths, have been reported in individuals using
   ephedra-containing products. These concerns led to regulatory
   actions in many countries.
3. **Regulatory Restrictions:** Due to safety concerns, several countries, including the United States, Canada, and others, have implemented restrictions on the sale and use of dietary supplements
   containing ephedrine alkaloids.

Legal Status

1. **United States:** The U.S. Food and Drug Administration (FDA)
   banned the sale of dietary supplements containing ephedrine alkaloids in 2004. The ban was implemented due to concerns about
   the potential health risks associated with ephedra use.
2. **Other Countries:** Many other countries have also restricted or

banned the sale of ephedra-containing supplements due to safety concerns.

Herbal Medicine and Ephedra-Free Alternatives

1. **Herbal Alternatives:** In traditional herbal medicine, other herbs with stimulant properties, such as ginseng or green tea, may be considered as alternatives to ephedra.
2. **Weight Loss and Energy Supplements:** In the market, there are many weight-loss and energy supplements that do not contain ephedrine alkaloids. These typically use alternative ingredients and formulations.

Caution and Consultation

1. **Health Risks:** Due to the potential health risks associated with ephedra, individuals should exercise caution and avoid the use of products containing ephedrine alkaloids.
2. **Healthcare Professional Consultation:** If individuals are considering supplements for weight loss or energy, or if they have concerns about potential interactions with existing health conditions or medications, it is advisable to consult with a healthcare professional before using such products.

It's crucial to note that while ephedra has historical use in traditional medicine, its safety has come into question, leading to regulatory actions in various regions. Individuals should prioritize their health and well-being and seek guidance from healthcare professionals when considering the use of supplements or herbal products.

Brahmi

Brahmi, scientifically known as Bacopa monnieri, is a herb that has been used in traditional Ayurvedic medicine for centuries. It is known for its potential cognitive and adaptogenic properties. Here are some key points about Brahmi:

Botanical Description

1. **Plant Characteristics:** Brahmi is a creeping herb that grows in wetlands and is native to India, North America, Europe, Australia, and Asia.
2. **Leaves:** The leaves of the Brahmi plant are small, succulent, and oblong. They are often used for their medicinal properties.

Traditional Uses

1. **Ayurvedic Medicine:** Brahmi has a long history of use in Ayurvedic medicine, where it is considered a "Medhya Rasayana," a substance that enhances memory, intellect, and overall brain function.
2. **Memory Enhancement:** Brahmi is traditionally used to improve memory, cognitive function, and concentration. It is often used as a brain tonic.
3. **Stress and Anxiety:** Brahmi is known for its adaptogenic properties, helping the body adapt to stress. It may have a calming effect on the mind, and it is sometimes used to manage stress and anxiety.
4. **Other Traditional Uses:** In Ayurveda, Brahmi is also used for various purposes, including promoting healthy skin, supporting the nervous system, and improving digestive function.

Active Compounds

1. **Bacosides:** The primary active compounds in Brahmi are bacosides, which are believed to contribute to its cognitive-enhancing effects. Bacosides may have neuroprotective and antioxidant properties.

Modern Research

1. **Cognitive Function:** Some research studies suggest that Brahmi may have positive effects on cognitive function, memory, and

learning. It is believed to support the production of certain neurotransmitters in the brain.

2. **Anxiety and Stress:** There is evidence suggesting that Brahmi may have anxiolytic (anxiety-reducing) effects and may help in managing stress. It is thought to modulate the activity of certain neurotransmitters.

Forms of Consumption

1. **Herbal Supplements:** Brahmi is commonly available in the form of herbal supplements, including capsules, tablets, and liquid extracts.
2. **Tea and Infusions:** Brahmi leaves can be used to make herbal teas or infusions. This is a traditional method of consumption.

Precautions and Considerations

1. **Pregnancy and Breastfeeding:** Pregnant or breastfeeding women should exercise caution, and it is advisable to consult with a healthcare professional before using Brahmi supplements.
2. **Potential Interactions:** Individuals taking medications or having pre-existing health conditions should consult with a healthcare provider before using Brahmi, as it may interact with certain medications.

Dosage

1. **Dosage Recommendations:** The appropriate dosage of Brahmi can vary, and it is advisable to follow the recommended dosage on the product label or consult with a healthcare professional for personalized advice.

Conclusion

Brahmi is a herb with a rich history in traditional medicine, particularly in Ayurveda. While it has been traditionally used for cognitive

enhancement and stress management, individual responses may vary. If considering Brahmi supplements for specific health goals, it is recommended to consult with a healthcare professional to ensure safety and appropriateness, especially considering potential interactions with medications and individual health conditions.

Ginkgo Biloba

Ginkgo biloba is a popular herbal supplement derived from the leaves of the Ginkgo biloba tree, one of the oldest tree species on Earth. Ginkgo biloba has been used in traditional medicine for centuries, and it is known for its potential cognitive and circulatory benefits. Here are some key points about Ginkgo biloba:

Key Components

1. **Flavonoids and Terpenoids:** Ginkgo biloba leaves contain bioactive compounds, including flavonoids and terpenoids. These compounds have antioxidant properties.
2. **Ginkgolides and Bilobalide:** Ginkgo leaves also contain unique compounds known as ginkgolides and bilobalide, which are believed to have various physiological effects.

Traditional Uses

1. **Cognitive Function:** Ginkgo biloba has been traditionally used to support cognitive function, including memory and concentration. It is often promoted as a memory enhancer.
2. **Peripheral Circulation:** The herb is believed to improve blood circulation, particularly in the extremities, and it is sometimes used to alleviate symptoms associated with poor circulation.

Modern Research

1. **Cognitive Benefits:** Some studies suggest that Ginkgo biloba may have mild cognitive-enhancing effects, especially in individu-

als with age-related cognitive decline. However, results have been mixed, and more research is needed.

2. **Peripheral Arterial Disease (PAD):** Ginkgo biloba has been investigated for its potential benefits in managing symptoms of peripheral arterial disease, such as leg pain during walking. Some studies suggest modest improvements.

3. **Antioxidant Properties:** Ginkgo biloba's flavonoids and ter-penoids have antioxidant properties, which may help protect cells from oxidative stress.

Forms of Consumption

1. **Dietary Supplements:** Ginkgo biloba is commonly available in the form of dietary supplements, including capsules, tablets, and liquid extracts.

2. **Tea:** Some people prepare Ginkgo biloba tea by infusing the dried leaves in hot water.

Precautions and Considerations

1. **Blood Thinning:** Ginkgo biloba has blood-thinning properties, and it may interact with anticoagulant medications. Individuals taking blood-thinning medications should consult with a health-care professional before using Ginkgo biloba.

2. **Side Effects:** While Ginkgo biloba is generally well-tolerated, some individuals may experience side effects, such as gastrointestinal discomfort or headaches. If adverse reactions occur, it is advisable to discontinue use.

3. **Pregnancy and Breastfeeding:** Pregnant or breastfeeding individuals should consult with a healthcare provider before using Ginkgo biloba supplements.

4. **Allergies:** Individuals with allergies to Ginkgo biloba or related plants should avoid its use.

Dosage

1. **Dosage Recommendations:** Dosages can vary, and it is important to follow the recommended dosage on the product label or consult with a healthcare professional for personalized advice.

Conclusion

Ginkgo biloba is a widely used herbal supplement with a long history of traditional use. While it is often promoted for cognitive benefits and improved circulation, its efficacy remains a subject of ongoing research. As with any dietary supplement, individuals should exercise caution, especially if they have underlying health conditions or are taking medications. Consulting with a healthcare professional is recommended to ensure the appropriateness and safety of Ginkgo biloba supplementation.

Ashwagandha

Ashwagandha, scientifically known as Withania somnifera, is an adaptogenic herb that has been used for centuries in traditional Ayurvedic medicine. It is native to the Indian subcontinent and is also known by other names, including Indian ginseng or winter cherry. Here are some key points about Ashwagandha:

Adaptogenic Properties

1. **Adaptogen Definition:** Adaptogens are substances that may help the body adapt to stress and promote overall well-being. Ashwagandha is classified as an adaptogen in traditional herbal medicine.
2. **Stress Management:** Ashwagandha is traditionally used to help the body cope with stress and promote a sense of balance. It is believed to have a calming effect on the nervous system.

Active Compounds

1. **Withanolides:** The primary active compounds in Ashwagandha are called withanolides. These compounds are believed to contribute to the herb's adaptogenic and medicinal properties.

Traditional Uses

1. **Energy and Vitality:** In Ayurvedic medicine, Ashwagandha is used to enhance vitality, energy, and overall well-being. It is sometimes referred to as a "rasayana" or rejuvenating herb.
2. **Cognitive Function:** Ashwagandha is traditionally believed to support cognitive function, including memory and concentration.
3. **Immune System Support:** Some traditional uses include supporting the immune system and promoting overall immune health.
4. **Reproductive Health:** In Ayurveda, Ashwagandha has been used to support reproductive health in both men and women. It is considered a tonic for the reproductive system.

Modern Research

1. **Stress Reduction:** Some scientific studies suggest that Ashwagandha may help reduce stress and anxiety levels. It is believed to modulate the stress response in the body.
2. **Cognitive Benefits:** There is ongoing research on Ashwagandha's potential cognitive benefits, including its neuroprotective effects.
3. **Anti-Inflammatory Properties:** Ashwagandha is thought to have anti-inflammatory properties, which may contribute to its overall health benefi

Forms of Consumption

1. **Dietary Supplements:** Ashwagandha is commonly available in the form of dietary supplements, including capsules, tablets, and powder. Standardized extracts are often used to ensure consistent levels of active compounds.
2. **Ayurvedic Formulations:** In Ayurvedic practice, Ashwagandha

is sometimes used in combination with other herbs in specific formulations.

Dosage

1. **Dosage Recommendations:** The appropriate dosage of Ashwagandha can vary, and it is advisable to follow the recommended dosage on the product label or consult with a healthcare professional for personalized advice.

Precautions and Considerations

1. **Pregnancy and Breastfeeding:** Pregnant or breastfeeding individuals should consult with a healthcare provider before using Ashwagandha supplements.
2. **Interactions with Medications:** Individuals taking medications or having pre-existing health conditions should consult with a healthcare professional before using Ashwagandha, as it may interact with certain medications.
3. **Allergies:** Individuals with allergies to plants in the Solanaceae family (e.g., tomatoes, potatoes) should exercise caution, as Ashwagandha belongs to this plant family.

Conclusion

Ashwagandha is a well-regarded herb in traditional medicine, and its popularity has grown in modern times. While scientific research supports some of its traditional uses, individuals should be mindful of their health status and consult with healthcare professionals before incorporating Ashwagandha supplements, especially if they have specific health concerns or are taking medications.

Sweet Flag

Sweet flag, scientifically known as Acorus calamus, is a perennial herbaceous plant that is native to marshy areas in Europe, Asia, and

North America. It is also known by other names, including calamus or flagroot. Here are some key points about sweet flag:

Botanical Description

1. **Appearance:** Sweet flag typically grows in wet or marshy environments and has long, narrow, sword-like leaves that emerge from a central base.
2. **Rhizomes:** The underground stems, known as rhizomes, are the part of the plant that is commonly used for various purposes.

Traditional Uses

1. **Traditional Medicine:** Sweet flag has a long history of use in traditional medicine systems, including Ayurveda and traditional Chinese medicine (TCM).
2. **Digestive Aid:** In traditional herbal medicine, sweet flag has been used to support digestion. It is believed to have carminative properties, meaning it may help alleviate digestive discomfort.
3. **Cognitive Support:** Sweet flag has been traditionally associated with cognitive support and mental clarity. It is believed to have a calming effect on the mind.
4. **Aromatic Properties:** The rhizomes of sweet flag have a distinct aromatic scent and are sometimes used to add fragrance to herbal formulations.

Active Compounds

1. **Acorus Oil:** The essential oil derived from sweet flag contains several compounds, including β-asarone, which is believed to contribute to its properties.

Modern Research

1. **Pharmacological Properties:** Sweet flag has been studied for its pharmacological properties, including its potential effects on the nervous system and digestive system.
2. **CNS Effects:** Some studies have explored the effects of sweet flag on the central nervous system (CNS), suggesting potential neuroprotective and cognitive-enhancing properties. However, more research is needed in this area.
3. **Antimicrobial Activity:** Sweet flag has demonstrated antimicrobial properties in some studies, which may contribute to its traditional use for digestive support.

Forms of Consumption

1. **Herbal Preparations:** Sweet flag is available in various forms, including herbal preparations, tinctures, and essential oil.
2. **Chewing:** In some cultures, people have chewed on the rhizomes of sweet flag for their aromatic and potential digestive benefits.

Precautions and Considerations

1. **β-Asarone Content:** One compound found in sweet flag, β-asarone, has been a subject of concern due to potential toxicity. Some varieties of sweet flag may contain higher levels of β-asarone, which has led to regulatory restrictions in certain regions.
2. **Regulatory Status:** In some countries, the sale of sweet flag products is regulated due to concerns about β-asarone content. It is essential to be aware of the regulatory status in your region.
3. **Pregnancy and Lactation:** Due to the concerns about β-asarone, pregnant and breastfeeding individuals are generally advised to avoid the use of sweet flag.
4. **Individual Variability:** Responses to sweet flag can vary among individuals, and excessive consumption may lead to adverse effects. It is advisable to use it under the guidance of a qualified healthcare professional.

Conclusion

Sweet flag has a history of traditional use for digestive support and cognitive benefits. However, concerns about the presence of β-asarone have led to regulatory considerations. If considering the use of sweet flag for specific purposes, it is advisable to consult with a qualified healthcare professional and be aware of regulatory restrictions in your area

Rhodiola Rosea

Rhodiola rosea, commonly known as golden root or Arctic root, is a perennial herb that belongs to the Crassulaceae family. It is native to the mountainous regions of Europe, Asia, and North America. Rhodiola has been used for centuries in traditional medicine, particularly in Russia and Scandinavia. Here are some key points about Rhodiola rosea:

Adaptogenic Properties

1. **Adaptogen Definition:** Rhodiola rosea is classified as an adaptogen—a substance that is believed to help the body adapt to stress and promote overall well-being.
2. **Stress Response:** Rhodiola is traditionally used to enhance resilience to stress and reduce fatigue. It is believed to modulate the body's stress response and support balance.

Active Compounds

1. **Rosavins and Salidroside:** Rhodiola rosea contains bioactive compounds, including rosavins and salidroside. These compounds are believed to contribute to its adaptogenic effects.

Traditional Uses

1. **Energy and Endurance:** Rhodiola is traditionally used to combat fatigue, increase energy levels, and enhance physical and mental endurance.

2. **Cognitive Function:** It is believed to have cognitive-enhancing properties, including potential benefits for memory and concentration.
3. **Mood Support:** Rhodiola has been used traditionally to support mood and alleviate symptoms of mild to moderate depression.

Modern Research

1. **Adaptogenic Effects:** Some scientific studies support the adaptogenic properties of Rhodiola, suggesting its potential to improve stress resilience and reduce fatigue.
2. **Cognitive Function:** Research has explored Rhodiola's impact on cognitive function, including memory and attention. It may have neuroprotective effects.
3. **Physical Performance:** There is some evidence suggesting that Rhodiola may improve exercise performance and reduce perceived exertion during physical activities.
4. **Mood and Stress Reduction:** Rhodiola has been studied for its potential role in reducing symptoms of stress, anxiety, and mild to moderate depression.

Forms of Consumption

1. **Dietary Supplements:** Rhodiola rosea is commonly available in the form of dietary supplements, including capsules, tablets, and liquid extracts.
2. **Tea:** Some people prepare Rhodiola tea by infusing the dried root in hot water, although this method is less common than using supplements.

Dosage

1. **Dosage Recommendations:** The appropriate dosage of Rhodiola can vary, and it is advisable to follow the recommended dosage on the product label or consult with a healthcare professional for personalized advice.

Precautions and Considerations

1. **Individual Variability:** Responses to Rhodiola can vary among individuals. Some people may experience side effects, such as insomnia or jitteriness, especially if taken in high doses.
2. **Interactions:** Rhodiola may interact with certain medications, such as antidepressants and stimulants. Individuals taking medications should consult with a healthcare professional before using Rhodiola supplements.
3. **Pregnancy and Breastfeeding:** Pregnant or breastfeeding individuals should exercise caution, and it is advisable to consult with a healthcare provider before using Rhodiola

Conclusion

Rhodiola rosea is a well-regarded adaptogenic herb with a history of traditional use. While research supports some of its potential benefits, individual responses can vary. If considering the use of Rhodiola supplements for specific health goals, it is recommended to consult with a qualified healthcare professional, especially if there are pre-existing health conditions or concerns about potential interactions with medications.

ESUMA

Suma, scientifically known as Pfaffia paniculata, is a flowering plant native to the Amazon rainforest in South America. Also known as Brazilian ginseng, Suma has been used in traditional medicine by indigenous people in the Amazon basin for various health purposes. Here are some key points about Suma:

Traditional Uses

1. **Adaptogenic Properties:** Suma is considered an adaptogen, which means it is believed to help the body adapt to stress and promote overall well-being. It has a long history of traditional use by indigenous tribes in the Amazon for its adaptogenic properties.

2. **Energy and Vitality:** Suma has been traditionally used to increase energy levels, improve vitality, and combat fatigue. It is often referred to as "para todo" in South America, which translates to "for all" or "for everything."

3. **Immune Support:** In traditional medicine, Suma has been used to support the immune system and promote overall health.

Active Compounds

1. **Ecdysteroids:** Suma contains bioactive compounds known as ecdysteroids, which are believed to contribute to its adaptogenic and potential physiological effects.

2. **Pfaffosides:** Specific compounds called pfaffosides have been identified in Suma and may have antioxidant properties.

Modern Research

1. **Adaptogenic Effects:** While Suma has a history of traditional use, scientific research on its adaptogenic effects and other potential health benefits is limited compared to some other adaptogenic herbs.

Forms of Consumption

1. **Dietary Supplements:** Suma is commonly available in the form of dietary supplements, including capsules, tablets, and liquid extracts.

Dosage

1. **Dosage Recommendations:** The appropriate dosage of Suma can vary, and it is advisable to follow the recommended dosage on the product label or consult with a healthcare professional for personalized advice.

Precautions and Considerations

1. **Individual Variability:** Responses to Suma can vary among individuals. As with any herbal supplement, it's important to start with a lower dose and monitor for any potential adverse reactions.
2. **Interactions:** While Suma is generally considered safe, individuals taking medications or with pre-existing health conditions should consult with a healthcare professional before using Suma supplements to avoid potential interactions.
3. **Pregnancy and Breastfeeding:** Pregnant or breastfeeding individuals should exercise caution, and it is advisable to consult with a healthcare provider before using Suma.
4. **Allergies:** Individuals with allergies to plants in the Amaranthaceae family (such as quinoa or beets) should exercise caution, as Suma belongs to this plant family.

Conclusion

Suma is a plant with a history of traditional use in the Amazon rainforest, and it is valued for its adaptogenic properties. While it is generally considered safe, scientific research on its specific effects is limited. Individuals considering the use of Suma supplements should approach it with caution, especially if they have pre-existing health conditions or are taking medications. Consulting with a healthcare professional is advisable for personalized guidance.

Betel Nut

Betel nut, also known as areca nut, is the seed of the Areca catechu palm tree. It is commonly chewed for its stimulant properties in many Asian and Pacific regions, and it plays a significant cultural and social role in certain communities. Here are some key points about betel nut:

Cultural and Traditional Use

1. **Chewing Tradition:** Betel nut chewing is a cultural and social practice in various Asian and Pacific countries. It is often wrapped

in a betel leaf along with slaked lime (calcium hydroxide) and other additives.

2. **Stimulant Effects:** Betel nut contains alkaloids, particularly arecoline, which has stimulant properties. Chewing betel nut can lead to increased alertness, heightened mood, and a mild euphoric effect.

3. **Social and Ritualistic Use:** The practice of betel nut chewing is deeply embedded in social and cultural rituals. It is often offered as a gesture of hospitality and used in ceremonies and celebrations.

Active Compounds

1. **Arecoline:** Arecoline is the primary alkaloid found in betel nut and is responsible for its stimulant effects. It acts on the central nervous system, similar to nicotine.

Health Concerns

1. **Oral Health Issues:** Prolonged and frequent betel nut chewing has been associated with various oral health issues, including stained teeth, gum problems, and an increased risk of oral cancer.

2. **Carcinogenicity:** The International Agency for Research on Cancer (IARC) classifies betel quid (betel nut, betel leaf, and slaked lime) as a Group 1 human carcinogen, indicating there is sufficient evidence to support its carcinogenicity, particularly with regard to oral cancers.

3. **Addiction Potential:** Regular use of betel nut has the potential for dependence, and cessation may lead to withdrawal symptoms.

Regulation and Legal Status

1. **Regulation:** The sale and use of betel nut are regulated in some countries due to its health concerns and potential for abuse.

2. **Bans:** In certain regions, there are restrictions or outright bans on the sale and consumption of betel nut. These measures aim to address public health issues associated with its use.

Betel Quid and Associated Risks

1. **Betel Quid:** Betel quid refers to a combination of betel nut, betel leaf, slaked lime, and sometimes tobacco. The combination of these ingredients contributes to the potential health risks associated with betel quid chewing.
2. **Public Health Campaigns:** Public health campaigns in some countries aim to raise awareness about the health risks of betel quid chewing and encourage cessation.

Conclusion

While betel nut chewing has cultural significance and is deeply rooted in certain traditions, it is important to be aware of the associated health risks. The practice has been linked to various oral health issues and an increased risk of certain cancers. Individuals should consider the potential health implications before engaging in betel nut chewing, and public health efforts often focus on education and prevention to address the risks associated with this practice. If there are concerns about betel nut use and its impact on health, seeking guidance from healthcare professionals is advisable.

Agrimony

Agrimony refers to a genus of herbaceous flowering plants belonging to the rose family (Rosaceae). The most commonly known species within this genus is Agrimonia eupatoria, also known as common agrimony or church steeples. Here are some key points about agrimony:

Botanical Description

1. **Appearance:** Agrimony plants typically have slender stems, compound leaves, and small yellow flowers arranged in spikes.
2. **Habitat:** They are commonly found in meadows, fields, and woodland edges, and they are native to Europe and Asia.

Traditional Uses

1. **Herbal Medicine:** Agrimony has a long history of use in traditional herbal medicine. The leaves, flowers, and roots are often used in herbal preparations.
2. **Digestive Aid:** Agrimony is traditionally used to support digestive health. It is believed to have astringent properties that may help with mild gastrointestinal issues.
3. **Topical Use:** In traditional herbal remedies, agrimony has been used topically for skin conditions and wounds. It is sometimes applied as a poultice.

Active Compounds

1. **Tannins:** Agrimony contains tannins, which are polyphenolic compounds with astringent properties. Tannins are believed to contribute to agrimony's potential medicinal effects.
2. **Flavonoids:** Flavonoids are also present in agrimony and may contribute to its antioxidant properties.

Modern Research

1. **Limited Studies:** While agrimony has a history of traditional use, there is limited modern scientific research on its specific therapeutic effects. More research is needed to establish its efficacy and safety.

Forms of Consumption

1. **Herbal Tea:** Agrimony leaves and flowers are sometimes used to prepare herbal teas. The tea is often consumed for its potential digestive benefits.
2. **Herbal Extracts and Tinctures:** Agrimony extracts and tinctures are available in some herbal formulations.

Precautions and Considerations

1. **Allergies:** Individuals with known allergies to plants in the rose family (Rosaceae) should exercise caution when using agrimony.
2. **Pregnancy and Breastfeeding:** Pregnant or breastfeeding individuals should consult with a healthcare professional before using agrimony products.
3. **Medical Conditions and Medications:** People with pre-existing health conditions or those taking medications should seek advice from a healthcare provider before using agrimony supplements due to potential interactions.

Conclusion

Agrimony is a traditional herb that has been used for various purposes, especially in the context of traditional herbal medicine. While it is generally considered safe when used appropriately, individuals should be aware of potential interactions and consult with healthcare professionals, especially if they have specific health concerns or are taking medications. As with any herbal remedy, it's important to approach its use with caution and consider the available scientific evidence.

Alder

Alder refers to a genus of deciduous trees and shrubs belonging to the family Betulaceae. The most well-known species within this genus is Alnus glutinosa, commonly known as European alder. Here are some key points about alder:

Botanical Description

1. **Leaves:** Alder leaves are alternate, simple, and serrated. They are usually dark green and somewhat rounded.
2. **Catkins:** Like many trees in the Betulaceae family, alders produce catkins. Male catkins are long and pendulous, while female catkins are smaller and more inconspicuous.

3. **Bark:** The bark of alder trees is typically smooth and grayish-brown when young, becoming rougher and darker with age.

Common Species

1. **European Alder (Alnus glutinosa):** Native to Europe, it is often found in wetland habitats and is known for its association with waterlogged soils.
2. **Red Alder (Alnus rubra):** Native to western North America, red alder is commonly found in riparian areas and is known for its nitrogen-fixing abilities.
3. **White Alder (Alnus rhombifolia):** Native to western North America, white alder is found in riparian habitats and has distinctive diamond-shaped leaves.

Ecological Importance

1. **Nitrogen Fixation:** Alders are nitrogen-fixing trees, which means they have a symbiotic relationship with nitrogen-fixing bacteria in their root nodules. This ability contributes to soil fertility.
2. **Habitat Support:** Alders are often found in wetland habitats, and their presence can contribute to habitat diversity and stability.

Uses

1. **Wood:** Alder wood is light in color and relatively soft. It is used for various purposes, including furniture, cabinets, and woodcraft.
2. **Landscaping:** Alder trees are sometimes planted for landscaping purposes, especially in wet areas, to stabilize soils and provide habitat.
3. **Traditional Uses:** Historically, various parts of the alder tree, including the bark and leaves, have been used in traditional medicine for various purposes.

Environmental Considerations

1. **Restoration:** Due to their nitrogen-fixing ability and adaptability to wetland conditions, alders are sometimes used in ecological restoration projects to improve soil quality.
2. **Invasive Potential:** In some regions, certain alder species may have invasive tendencies, disrupting local ecosystems.

Conclusion

Alder trees are valued for their ecological role, especially in wetland habitats, and have practical uses such as wood production. While they have been used historically for certain traditional purposes, individuals should exercise caution and seek proper guidance if considering the use of alder products for medicinal or other purposes. Additionally, the potential invasive nature of certain alder species in specific regions should be considered in ecological contexts

Aloe

Aloe refers to a genus of succulent plants that includes over 500 species. The most commonly known species is Aloe vera, also known as true aloe or medicinal aloe. Here are some key points about aloe, particularly Aloe vera:

Botanical Description

1. **Appearance:** Aloe plants typically have thick, fleshy leaves arranged in a rosette pattern. The leaves often have serrated edges and contain a gel-like substance.
2. **Flowers:** Aloe plants produce tubular flowers on tall stalks, usually in shades of red, orange, or yellow.

Aloe Vera

1. **Common Name:** Aloe vera is commonly known as true aloe, medicinal aloe, or simply aloe.
2. **Gel:** The inner gel of Aloe vera leaves is widely recognized for its soothing and moisturizing properties. It is commonly used in various skincare and cosmetic products.
3. **Latex:** A yellowish substance called aloe latex can be found just beneath the skin of the Aloe vera leaf. It contains compounds with potential laxative effects.

Traditional Uses

1. **Skin Care:** Aloe vera gel has a long history of traditional use for skin care. It is applied topically to soothe and moisturize the skin and may be used for minor burns, cuts, and irritations.
2. **Digestive Health:** Aloe latex, derived from the inner leaf skin, has been traditionally used for its potential laxative effects. However, its use as a laxative is not recommended without proper supervision due to concerns about safety and potential side effects.

Modern Uses

1. **Skincare Products:** Aloe vera is a common ingredient in a variety of skincare products, including lotions, creams, and sunburn relief gels.
2. **Digestive Supplements:** Aloe latex is sometimes used in dietary supplements for its potential laxative properties. However, its use for this purpose is controversial, and it is not recommended without medical supervision.

Health Considerations

1. **Topical Use:** Aloe vera gel is generally considered safe for topical use. It is well-tolerated by many individuals and is used to promote skin hydration and alleviate minor skin irritations.
2. **Oral Use:** Internal use of aloe products, especially those containing

aloe latex, should be approached with caution. Aloe latex may have potential side effects, and its use as a laxative is not recommended without proper guidance from a healthcare professional.

3. **Pregnancy and Breastfeeding:** Pregnant or breastfeeding individuals should exercise caution with internal use of aloe products and consult with a healthcare provider.

Conclusion

Aloe vera is a versatile plant with a long history of traditional use, particularly for skincare. When used topically, aloe vera gel is generally safe and well-tolerated. However, internal use, especially of aloe latex, requires caution and should be done under the guidance of a healthcare professional due to potential side effects. As with any plant-based product, individual reactions can vary, and it's important to be aware of potential contraindications and interactions with medications.

Balsam Root

Balsam root typically refers to plants belonging to the Balsamorhiza genus, particularly Balsamorhiza sagittata, which is commonly known as arrowleaf balsamroot. Here are some key points about balsam root:

Botanical Description

1. **Appearance:** Arrowleaf balsamroot is a perennial herb with large, arrow-shaped leaves. The plant typically reaches a height of 1 to 3 feet.
2. **Flowers:** The plant produces bright yellow, sunflower-like flowers with a prominent central disk. The flowers are borne on tall stems and bloom in late spring to early summer.

Habitat and Distribution

1. **Native Range:** Arrowleaf balsamroot is native to western North America, and it is commonly found in a variety of habitats, including grasslands, prairies, and open woodlands.
2. **Adaptability:** Balsam root is adapted to various soil types and can thrive in different elevations and environmental conditions.

Traditional Uses

1. **Food Source:** Indigenous peoples of North America have traditionally used balsam root as a food source. The starchy taproots were often harvested, dried, and ground into a flour for use in cooking.
2. **Medicinal Uses:** Various Native American tribes used parts of the balsam root plant for medicinal purposes. The root was sometimes used topically for skin conditions, and infusions were made for internal use.

Modern Uses

1. **Wildlife Habitat:** Balsam root provides habitat and food for wildlife, including insects, birds, and small mammals.
2. **Erosion Control:** The deep, fibrous roots of balsam root help stabilize soil, making it valuable for erosion control.

Conservation

1. **Native Plant Conservation:** Given its ecological importance and traditional uses, conservation efforts may focus on protecting and preserving native balsam root populations.

Conclusion

Arrowleaf balsamroot is a native plant of western North America with cultural significance and ecological importance. Its traditional uses by indigenous peoples highlight its versatility as a food source and medicinal plant. As with any plant, responsible and sustainable harvesting practices are crucial for conservation, and efforts may be made to protect and maintain populations of balsam root for future generations.

St. John's Wort

St. John's Wort (Hypericum perforatum) is a flowering plant with yellow, star-shaped flowers that has been used for centuries for various medicinal purposes. Here are some key points about St. John's Wort:

Botanical Description

1. **Flowers:** St. John's Wort has bright yellow flowers with distinctive black dots along the edges, giving it a perforated appearance. The flowers bloom in late spring and early summer.
2. **Leaves:** The leaves are opposite, oblong, and dotted with translucent glands.
3. **Habitat:** St. John's Wort is a hardy perennial plant that thrives in sunny locations, often found in meadows, fields, and along roadsides.

Traditional Uses

1. **Historical Use:** St. John's Wort has a long history of use in traditional medicine, dating back to ancient Greece.
2. **Mood and Emotional Well-being:** It has been traditionally used to alleviate symptoms of mild to moderate depression and improve mood.
3. **Wound Healing:** St. John's Wort has also been used topically for its potential wound-healing properties. The infused oil is applied to the skin to promote healing.

Active Compounds

1. **Hypericin and Hyperforin:** St. John's Wort contains bioactive compounds, including hypericin and hyperforin, which are believed to contribute to its pharmacological effects.

Modern Research

1. **Antidepressant Properties:** St. John's Wort has been studied for its potential antidepressant effects. Some research suggests that it may be effective for mild to moderate depression.
2. **Mechanism of Action:** The exact mechanism of action of St. John's Wort is not fully understood, but it is believed to involve the modulation of neurotransmitters in the brain.
3. **Topical Use:** While the topical use of St. John's Wort oil has been traditional, scientific evidence supporting its efficacy for wound healing is limited.

Forms of Consumption

1. **Dietary Supplements:** St. John's Wort is commonly available in the form of dietary supplements, including capsules, tablets, and liquid extracts.
2. **Topical Preparations:** Infused oils or creams containing St. John's Wort are sometimes used topically for skin conditions.

Precautions and Considerations

1. **Interaction with Medications:** St. John's Wort can interact with various medications, including antidepressants, birth control pills, and certain anticoagulants. It may reduce the effectiveness of these medications.
2. **Photosensitivity:** Some individuals may experience increased sensitivity to sunlight (photosensitivity) when taking St. John's Wort, leading to an increased risk of sunburn.
3. **Pregnancy and Breastfeeding:** Pregnant or breastfeeding

individuals should consult with a healthcare professional before using St. John's Wort due to potential risks.

4. **Side Effects:** While St. John's Wort is generally well-tolerated, some individuals may experience side effects such as gastrointestinal upset, dizziness, or skin reactions.

Conclusion

St. John's Wort is a widely studied herb with a history of traditional use for mood-related issues. While research supports its potential antidepressant effects, caution is necessary due to its interactions with medications. Individuals considering the use of St. John's Wort for specific health concerns should consult with a healthcare professional to ensure its appropriateness and safety, especially if they are taking other medications.

Marjoram

Marjoram (Origanum majorana) is a fragrant herb belonging to the mint family (Lamiaceae). It is closely related to oregano (Origanum vulgare) and is known for its aromatic leaves that are commonly used as a culinary herb. Here are some key points about marjoram:

Botanical Description

1. **Leaves:** Marjoram has small, oval-shaped leaves that are gray-green in color. The leaves are highly aromatic.
2. **Flowers:** The plant produces small clusters of white or pink flowers, typically in late spring to early summer.

Culinary Uses

1. **Flavor Profile:** Marjoram has a mild, sweet, and slightly floral flavor. It is often described as having a taste similar to oregano but milder.
2. **Culinary Applications:** Marjoram is a popular culinary herb

used in a variety of dishes, including soups, stews, sauces, dressings, and meat dishes. It pairs well with vegetables, poultry, and
seafood.

Medicinal Uses

1. **Traditional Medicine:** Marjoram has been used in traditional
   medicine for its potential medicinal properties. It was historically
   believed to have calming and digestive benefits.
2. **Aromatherapy:** The essential oil derived from marjoram is
   sometimes used in aromatherapy for its calming and soothing
   properties.

Growing Marjoram

1. **Cultivation:** Marjoram can be grown in gardens or containers.
   It prefers well-drained soil and full sunlight.
2. **Perennial Herb:** Marjoram is a perennial herb in warmer cli-
   mates but is often grown as an annual in cooler regions.

Nutritional Content

1. **Vitamins and Minerals:** While used primarily for its flavor,
   marjoram does contain some vitamins and minerals, including
   vitamin K, vitamin A, calcium, and iron.

Varieties

1. **Sweet Marjoram (Origanum majorana):** The most commonly
   cultivated variety used in culinary applications. It has a sweeter
   and milder flavor compared to oregano.
2. **Pot Marjoram (Origanum onites):** Another variety of marjoram, often used in cooking. It has a slightly different flavor profile
   than sweet marjoram.

Culinary Substitutes

1. **Oregano:** In some recipes, oregano can be used as a substitute for marjoram, although oregano has a stronger flavor.
2. **Thyme:** Thyme can also be used as a substitute for marjoram in certain dishes.

Conclusion

Marjoram is a versatile herb that adds a delightful flavor to a variety of dishes. Whether used fresh or dried, its aromatic and slightly sweet taste enhances the culinary experience. Beyond its culinary uses, marjoram has a history of traditional medicinal use, and its essential oil is valued in aromatherapy. Including marjoram in your herb garden or using it in cooking can bring a unique and pleasant flavor to your favorite dishes.

Wormwood

Wormwood refers to a genus of aromatic plants in the Artemisia family, with Artemisia absinthium being the most well-known species. Here are some key points about wormwood:

Botanical Description

1. **Leaves:** Wormwood has finely divided, silver-green leaves that are deeply lobed, giving the plant a feathery appearance.
2. **Flowers:** The plant produces small, yellow-green flowers in clusters.
3. **Aroma:** Wormwood is known for its strong and bitter aroma, which is attributed to the presence of essential oils.

Historical Uses

1. **Culinary Use:** Wormwood has historically been used in culinary applications, particularly in the production of absinthe, a highly

alcoholic and anise-flavored spirit. However, its use in food and beverages is regulated in many countries due to its potentially toxic compounds.

2. **Traditional Medicine:** Wormwood has been used in traditional medicine for various purposes, including as a digestive tonic and for its potential anti-parasitic properties. However, its use is associated with caution due to its strong constituents.

Active Compounds

1. **Thujone:** Wormwood contains thujone, a compound that is known for its neurotoxic effects in high doses. Thujone content is regulated in many countries due to concerns about its safety.
2. **Essential Oils:** Wormwood contains essential oils with compounds such as absinthin and anabsinthin, contributing to its bitter taste.

Modern Uses

1. **Beverage Production:** While wormwood has been historically used in the production of absinthe, modern regulations often limit the thujone content in absinthe.
2. **Herbal Preparations:** Wormwood is sometimes used in herbal formulations, but its use should be approached with caution due to the potential toxicity of thujone.

Precautions and Considerations

1. **Toxicity:** Wormwood, particularly its thujone content, can be toxic in high doses. Prolonged or excessive use should be avoided.
2. **Pregnancy and Breastfeeding:** Pregnant and breastfeeding individuals should avoid the use of wormwood due to its potential for harm.
3. **Neurological Effects:** Thujone can affect the central nervous system, leading to seizures and other adverse effects. It is important to adhere to recommended dosage guidelines.
4. **Regulatory Status:** The use of wormwood in food and beverag-

es is regulated in many countries due to concerns about thujone content.

Conclusion

Wormwood is a plant with a complex history, often associated with the production of absinthe and traditional medicine. Its bitter taste and potential toxicity, especially related to thujone, require caution in its use. The production and consumption of products containing wormwood are often subject to strict regulations to ensure safety. If considering the use of wormwood for any purpose, it is advisable to consult with healthcare professionals and adhere to regulatory guidelines.

Dandelion

Dandelion (Taraxacum officinale) is a common flowering plant that is well-known for its bright yellow flowers and distinctive fluffy seed heads. Despite being considered a weed in some contexts, dandelion has a variety of culinary and medicinal uses. Here are some key points about dandelion:

Botanical Description

1. **Leaves:** Dandelion leaves are deeply lobed, forming a rosette at the base of the plant. They are often toothed or jagged.
2. **Flowers:** Dandelion flowers are bright yellow and composed of numerous small florets. The flowers close at night and in cloudy weather.
3. **Seed Heads:** The characteristic fluffy seed heads are produced after flowering. Each seed is attached to a parachute-like structure that facilitates wind dispersal.

Culinary Uses

1. **Edible Leaves:** Dandelion leaves are edible and can be used in salads, sautéed, or added to soups. They have a slightly bitter taste.

2. **Roots:** Dandelion roots can be roasted and ground to make a caffeine-free coffee substitute. They have a rich, earthy flavor.
3. **Flowers:** The flowers can be used to make dandelion wine, and they are sometimes used in salads or for garnishing dishes.

Medicinal Uses

1. **Traditional Medicine:** Dandelion has a history of use in traditional medicine for various purposes, including as a diuretic and digestive aid.
2. **Detoxification:** Some herbal traditions use dandelion to support liver health and as a mild detoxifying agent.
3. **Nutrient Content:** Dandelion leaves are rich in vitamins and minerals, including vitamin A, vitamin C, and potassium.

Potential Health Benefits

1. **Diuretic Properties:** Dandelion has natural diuretic properties, which may help promote the excretion of excess fluids from the body.
2. **Antioxidant Content:** Dandelion contains antioxidants that may help neutralize free radicals in the body.
3. **Digestive Support:** Some people use dandelion to support digestive health, although more research is needed to confirm its efficacy for this purpose.

Forms of Consumption

1. **Tea:** Dandelion tea is a popular way to consume the plant. Both the leaves and roots can be used to make tea.
2. **Salads:** Young dandelion leaves can be added to salads or used in other culinary preparations.
3. **Supplements:** Dandelion supplements, including capsules and extracts, are available for those who prefer a more concentrated form.

Precautions and Considerations

1. **Foraging:** If foraging for dandelions, it's essential to ensure that they are sourced from areas free of pesticides and contaminants.
2. **Allergies:** Individuals with allergies to plants in the Asteraceae family (such as ragweed, marigolds, and chamomile) may also be allergic to dandelion.
3. **Interactions:** Dandelion supplements may interact with certain medications or medical conditions, so it's advisable to consult with a healthcare professional before using them.

Conclusion

Dandelion is a versatile plant with culinary and potential medicinal uses. While it's often considered a weed, many people appreciate its nutritional value and find creative ways to incorporate it into their diet. As with any herbal remedy, individuals should exercise caution, especially if considering the use of dandelion supplements, and consult with healthcare professionals if they have specific health concerns or are taking medications.

Chervil

Chervil (Anthriscus cerefolium) is a delicate, aromatic herb belonging to the parsley family (Apiaceae). It is native to Southern Europe and is known for its lacy, fern-like leaves and mild, anise-like flavor. Here are some key points about chervil:

Botanical Description

1. **Leaves:** Chervil leaves are finely divided, resembling fern fronds. The leaves are bright green and tender.
2. **Flowers:** Chervil produces small, white flowers arranged in umbrella-like clusters.

Culinary Uses

1. **Flavor Profile:** Chervil has a delicate, mild flavor with a hint of anise or licorice. It is often described as a cross between parsley and tarragon.
2. **Culinary Pairings:** Chervil is commonly used in French cuisine and pairs well with dishes such as salads, soups, sauces, and egg dishes. It is particularly popular in fines herbes, a classic French herb blend.
3. **Garnish:** Chervil is often used as a garnish, adding a touch of freshness to finished dishes.

Nutritional Content

1. **Vitamins and Minerals:** Chervil contains vitamins A and C, as well as minerals such as iron and potassium.

Growing Chervil

1. **Cultivation:** Chervil can be grown in gardens or containers. It prefers partial shade and moist, well-drained soil.
2. **Annual Herb:** Chervil is an annual herb, meaning it completes its life cycle within one growing season.

Harvesting

1. **Timing:** Chervil is best harvested when the leaves are young and tender, as the flavor can become stronger and the texture coarser as the plant matures.
2. **Use of Fresh Leaves:** Fresh chervil leaves are preferred in culinary applications, as they have the most delicate flavor.

Culinary Substitutes

1. **Parsley:** While not an exact match, parsley can be used as a substitute for chervil in recipes.

2. **Tarragon:** In some dishes, tarragon can provide a hint of anise flavor similar to chervil.

Medicinal Uses

1. **Traditional Medicine:** Chervil has been used in traditional medicine for various purposes, including as a digestive aid.
2. **Potential Health Benefits:** While chervil is primarily used for its culinary qualities, it contains certain compounds that may have mild antioxidant properties.

Precautions and Considerations

1. **Allergies:** Individuals with allergies to plants in the Apiaceae family (such as carrots, celery, and parsley) may also be sensitive to chervil.
2. **Pregnancy and Breastfeeding:** Pregnant or breastfeeding individuals should consult with a healthcare professional before using chervil in larger quantities.

Conclusion

Chervil is a versatile herb valued for its delicate flavor and aesthetic appeal. Whether used to enhance the flavor of dishes or as a garnish, chervil adds a touch of elegance to culinary creations. Its mild taste makes it a favorite in French cuisine, and it's a delightful herb to grow and use in home gardens or kitchens.

Spearmint

Spearmint (Mentha spicata) is a fragrant herb that belongs to the mint family (Lamiaceae). It is a popular culinary herb known for its refreshing, sweet, and slightly menthol flavor. Here are some key points about spearmint:

Botanical Description

1. **Leaves:** Spearmint has bright green, serrated leaves that are often covered in fine hairs, giving them a slightly fuzzy appearance.
2. **Flowers:** The plant produces small, pink or lilac-colored flowers arranged in spikes.

Culinary Uses

1. **Flavor Profile:** Spearmint has a milder and sweeter flavor compared to peppermint. It is often described as having a clean, refreshing taste with a hint of sweetness.
2. **Culinary Applications:** Spearmint is widely used in both sweet and savory dishes. It is a key ingredient in mint sauces, salads, beverages (such as mint tea and mojitos), desserts, and as a garnish.
3. **Beverages:** Spearmint is commonly used to flavor various beverages, including teas, lemonades, and cocktails.

Medicinal Uses

1. **Digestive Aid:** Spearmint has been traditionally used to aid digestion. Mint teas, including spearmint tea, are often consumed for their digestive properties.
2. **Aromatherapy:** The aroma of spearmint is often used in aromatherapy for its refreshing and invigorating scent.

Growing Spearmint

1. **Cultivation:** Spearmint is a hardy perennial herb that grows well in a variety of conditions. It tends to spread quickly, so it's often grown in containers to control its growth.
2. **Sunlight and Soil:** Spearmint prefers partial to full sunlight and well-drained soil.

Varieties

1. **Common Spearmint (Mentha spicata):** The most widely cultivated variety with the characteristic sweet and mild flavor.
2. **Garden Mint:** Often used as a general term for spearmint varieties grown in home gardens.

Culinary Substitutes

1. **Peppermint:** While peppermint has a stronger and more menthol flavor, it can be used as a substitute for spearmint in certain recipes.
2. **Pennyroyal:** Another member of the mint family, pennyroyal, has a more intense flavor and should be used sparingly as a substitute.

Essential Oil

1. **Spearmint Essential Oil:** Extracted from the leaves of the spearmint plant, the essential oil is used in aromatherapy and for flavoring purposes.

Precautions and Considerations

1. **Invasive Growth:** Spearmint can be invasive and may take over garden spaces. Growing it in containers can help control its spread.
2. **Allergies:** Individuals with allergies to plants in the mint family should exercise caution when consuming spearmint.
3. **Pregnancy and Breastfeeding:** While moderate culinary use of spearmint is generally considered safe, excessive use of spearmint supplements may be avoided during pregnancy and breastfeeding.

Conclusion

Spearmint is a versatile herb widely appreciated for its culinary applications, refreshing flavor, and potential health benefits. Whether used in cooking, beverages, or aromatherapy, spearmint adds a delightful and aromatic touch to various experiences. Gardeners often enjoy growing spearmint for its easy cultivation and the joy it brings to the kitchen and garden.

Savory

Savory refers to a group of aromatic herbs in the genus Satureja, with two main varieties: summer savory (Satureja hortensis) and winter savory (Satureja montana). These herbs are known for their savory, slightly peppery flavor and are used in culinary applications. Here are some key points about savory:

Botanical Description

1. **Summer Savory (Satureja hortensis):**

    » **Annual Herb:** Summer savory is an annual herb, meaning it completes its life cycle in one growing season.
    » **Leaves:** The leaves of summer savory are small, narrow, and green, with a delicate texture.

2. **Winter Savory (Satureja montana):**

    » **Perennial Herb:** Winter savory is a perennial herb, meaning it can live for several years.
    » **Leaves:** Winter savory has darker green and more robust leaves compared to summer savory.

Culinary Uses

1. **Flavor Profile:** Savory has a pungent and peppery flavor, reminiscent of a cross between thyme and marjoram. It is often described as having a warming and earthy taste.
2. **Culinary Applications:** Both summer and winter savory are used in cooking, adding flavor to a variety of dishes. They are popular in meat dishes, stews, soups, vegetables, and herb blends.

3. **Drying:** Savory retains its flavor well when dried, making it a convenient herb to use in the kitchen throughout the year.

Growing Savory

1. **Cultivation:** Savory can be grown in gardens or containers. It prefers well-drained soil and full sunlight.
2. **Annual vs. Perennial:** Depending on the variety (summer or winter), savory can be grown as an annual or perennial herb.

Medicinal Uses

1. **Traditional Medicine:** Savory has been used in traditional medicine for various purposes, including as a digestive aid and to relieve respiratory issues.
2. **Antimicrobial Properties:** Some studies suggest that savory may have antimicrobial properties, contributing to its traditional use in supporting overall health.

Varieties

1. **Summer Savory (Satureja hortensis):** Commonly used in culinary applications and preferred for its delicate leaves.
2. **Winter Savory (Satureja montana):** Known for its hardier leaves and perennial growth habit.

Essential Oil

1. **Savory Essential Oil:** Extracted from the leaves of the savory plant, the essential oil is used in aromatherapy and sometimes for its potential health benefits.

Precautions and Considerations

1. **Pregnancy and Breastfeeding:** Pregnant or breastfeeding individuals should exercise caution with savory supplements and consult with a healthcare professional.
2. **Allergies:** Individuals with allergies to plants in the mint family (Lamiaceae) may also be sensitive to savory.
3. **Medical Conditions and Medications:** People with pre-existing health conditions or those taking medications should seek advice from a healthcare provider before using savory supplements.

Conclusion

Savory is a versatile herb with a robust flavor that enhances the taste of various dishes. Whether used fresh or dried, summer or winter savory, this herb contributes a distinct and savory quality to culinary creations. Gardeners and cooks alike appreciate the ease of cultivating and using savory in the kitchen.

Borage

Borage (Borago officinalis) is an annual herb with bright blue, star-shaped flowers. It is known for its culinary uses, medicinal properties, and its ability to attract pollinators. Here are some key points about borage:

Botanical Description

1. **Leaves:** Borage leaves are large, rough, and covered in fine, prickly hairs. They are typically oval or heart-shaped.
2. **Flowers:** Borage is known for its vibrant, blue flowers with five petals arranged in a star-like pattern. Pink and white varieties are also available.

Culinary Uses

1. **Flavor Profile:** Borage has a mild cucumber-like flavor, making its leaves and flowers suitable for culinary applications.
2. **Edible Flowers:** Both the leaves and flowers of borage are edible. The flowers are often used as a decorative element in salads, drinks, or desserts.
3. **Cooking:** Borage leaves can be used in salads, soups, or cooked as greens. The mild flavor complements a variety of dishes.

Medicinal Uses

1. **Traditional Medicine:** Borage has been used in traditional medicine for its potential anti-inflammatory properties and to support respiratory health.
2. **Rich in Gamma-Linolenic Acid (GLA):** Borage oil, extracted from the seeds, is a rich source of gamma-linolenic acid, an essential fatty acid with potential health benefits.

Growing Borage

1. **Cultivation:** Borage is easy to grow and often self-seeds. It thrives in well-drained soil and prefers full sunlight.
2. **Attracting Pollinators:** Borage is known for attracting bees and other pollinators to the garden, making it a beneficial companion plant.

Varieties

1. **Blue Borage (Borago officinalis):** The most common variety with vibrant blue flowers.
2. **White Borage:** A variety with white flowers, though less common than the blue form.

Other Uses

1. **Companion Planting:** Borage is often planted as a companion to other crops to enhance their growth and repel certain pests.
2. **Borage Tea:** Borage leaves can be used to make herbal tea, which is sometimes consumed for its potential calming effects.

Precautions and Considerations

1. **Prickly Hairs:** The leaves of borage can be prickly due to fine hairs, so handling with care is advised.
2. **Pregnancy:** Pregnant or breastfeeding individuals should exercise caution with borage supplements, and consulting with a healthcare professional is recommended.
3. **Allergies:** Individuals with allergies to plants in the Boraginaceae family (such as comfrey) may also be sensitive to borage.

Conclusion

Borage is a versatile herb valued for its culinary uses, attractive flowers, and potential medicinal benefits. Whether grown for its edible leaves and flowers, its role in companion planting, or its potential herbal applications, borage is a popular choice in home gardens. As with any herb, individuals should be aware of potential precautions and consider consulting healthcare professionals when incorporating borage into their diet or wellness routine.

Herbs aromatic

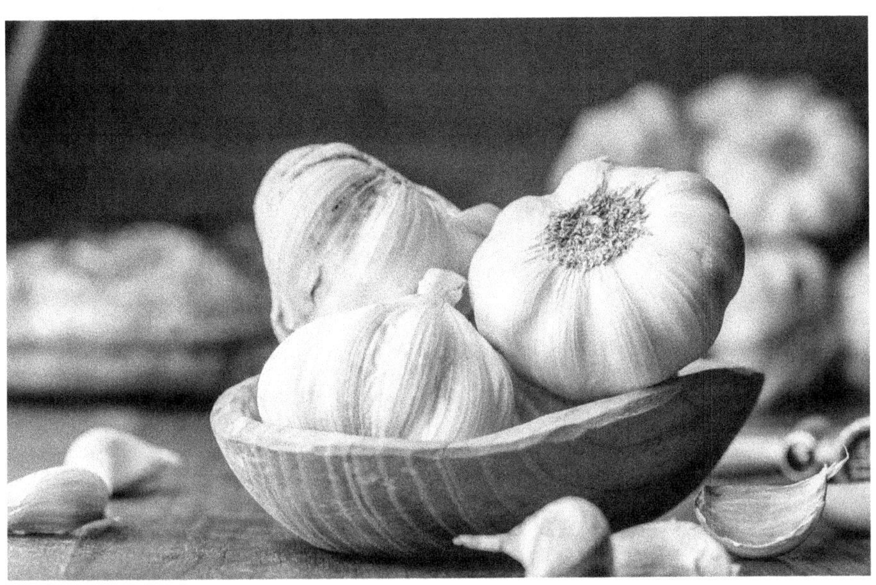

Garlic (Allium sativum)

Garlic is a bulbous plant known for its pungent flavor and aromatic qualities. It is widely used in various cuisines and is believed to have several health benefits.

Bay Leaf (Laurus nobilis)

Bay leaves come from the laurel tree and are used to add a subtle, aromatic flavor to soups, stews, and sauces. They are often dried before use.

Dill (Anethum graveolens)

Dill is a feathery herb with a fresh, anise-like flavor. It is commonly used in pickles, salads, and various dishes.

Basil (Ocimum basilicum)

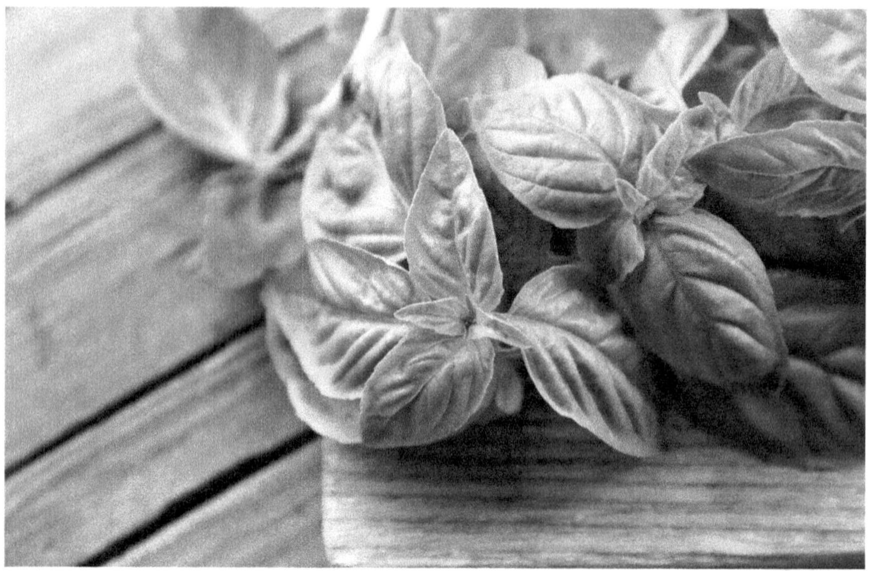

Basil is a fragrant herb with a sweet and slightly peppery flavor. It is a key ingredient in Italian cuisine and is often used in pesto.

Chervil (Anthriscus cerefolium)

Chervil has delicate, lacy leaves with a mild, anise-like flavor. It is used in salads, soups, and as a garnish.

Coriander (Coriandrum sativum)

Coriander, both the leaves (cilantro) and seeds, is used in various culinary dishes. It has a citrusy and slightly sweet taste.

Fennel (Foeniculum vulgare)

Fennel has a licorice-like flavor and is used in salads, as a vegetable, or to flavor dishes. The bulb, leaves, and seeds are all edible.

Lavender (Lavandula)

Lavender is known for its fragrant flowers. While it's commonly associated with aromatherapy and perfumes, culinary-grade lavender can be used in cooking and baking.

Marjoram (Origanum majorana)

Marjoram has a mild, sweet flavor and is often used in soups, stews, and meat dishes. It is a member of the oregano family.

Mint (Mentha)

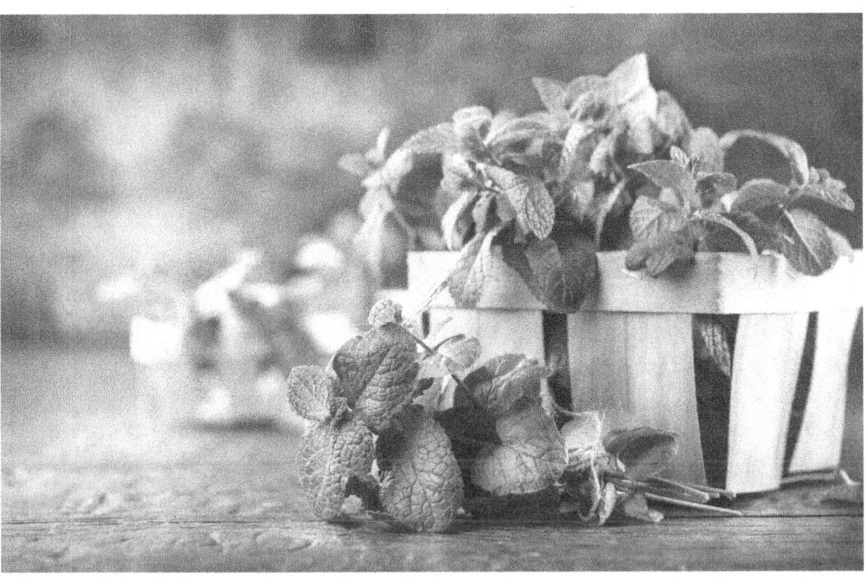

Mint is a refreshing herb with a cool, menthol flavor. It is used in beverages, desserts, and savory dishes.

Oregano (Origanum vulgare)

Oregano has a robust flavor and is a common herb in Mediterranean cuisine. It is used in pizza, pasta sauces, and meat dishes.

Parsley (Petroselinum crispum)

Parsley has a fresh, mild flavor and is used as a garnish or ingredient in a wide range of dishes, including salads and soups.

Rosemary (Rosmarinus officinalis)

Rosemary has a woody, aromatic flavor. It pairs well with roasted meats, potatoes, and in Mediterranean cuisine.

Sage (Salvia officinalis)

Sage has a slightly peppery flavor and is used in stuffing, savory dishes, and herbal teas. It has medicinal and culinary applications.

Savory (Satureja)

Savory, both summer and winter varieties, has a peppery taste and is used to season a variety of dishes, including beans, soups, and stews.

Celery (Apium graveolens)

Celery has a crisp texture and mild, slightly peppery flavor. It is used in salads, soups, and as a snack.

Thyme (Thymus vulgaris)

Thyme has a fragrant and earthy flavor. It is a versatile herb used in a wide range of dishes, from poultry to vegetables.

Tarragon (Artemisia dracunculus)

Tarragon has a distinct anise-like flavor and is used to flavor sauces, salads, and various dishes. It adds a unique twist to culinary creations.

Dragoncello (Artemisia dracunculus)

Dragoncello is another term for tarragon, known for its aromatic leaves and culinary uses.

Ginger (Zingiber officinale)

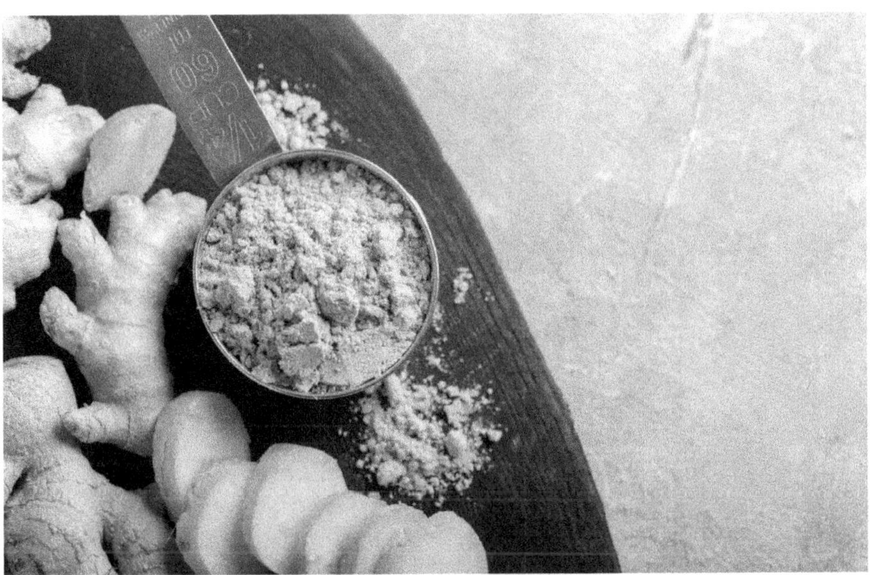

Ginger has a spicy and pungent flavor. It is used in both sweet and savory dishes, as well as in beverages. It is known for its medicinal properties.

CHAPTER 7

Herbs

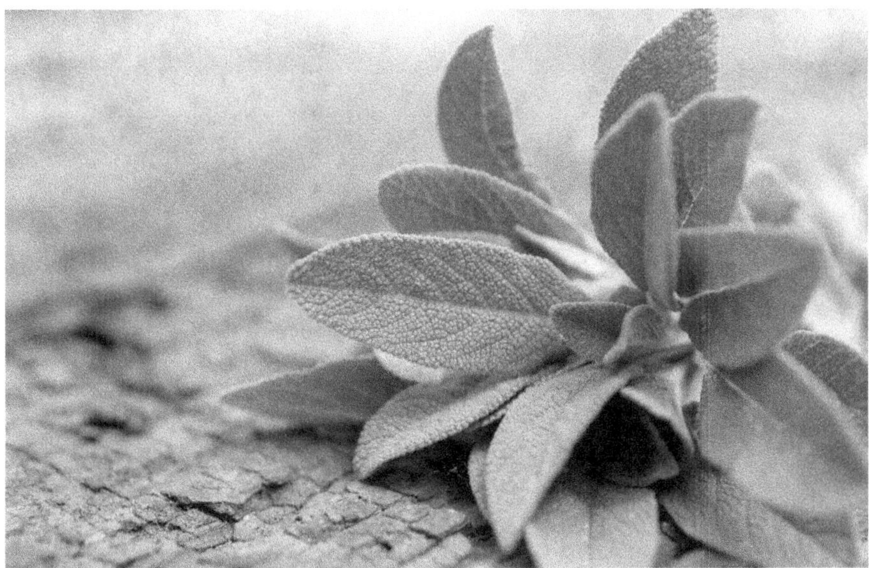

Sage (Salvia officinalis)

Sage is a fragrant herb with grayish-green leaves. It has a slightly peppery, earthy flavor and is often used in savory dishes, stuffing, and as a seasoning for meats.

Chamomile (Matricaria chamomilla)

Chamomile is a daisy-like flower with a mild, floral flavor. It is commonly used to make herbal tea, known for its calming and soothing properties.

Echinacea (Echinacea purpurea)

Echinacea is a medicinal herb known for its potential immune-boosting properties. It is often used in supplements and herbal teas.

Ginseng (Panax ginseng)

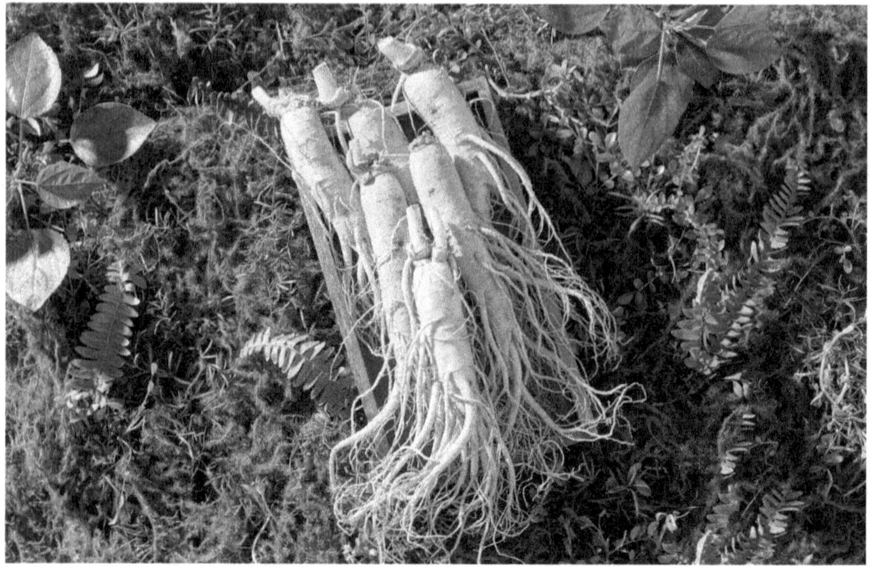

Ginseng is a root known for its adaptogenic properties. It is used in traditional medicine and supplements and is believed to provide energy and promote well-being.

Valerian (Valeriana officinalis)

Valerian is a herb with a strong, earthy aroma. It is commonly used as a natural remedy for sleep disorders and anxiety.

Mint (Mentha)

Mint is a refreshing herb with a cool, menthol flavor. It is used in beverages, desserts, and savory dishes.

Lavender (Lavandula)

Lavender is a fragrant flower often used in culinary applications and aromatherapy. It adds a floral note to dishes and is known for its calming scent.

Turmeric (Curcuma longa)

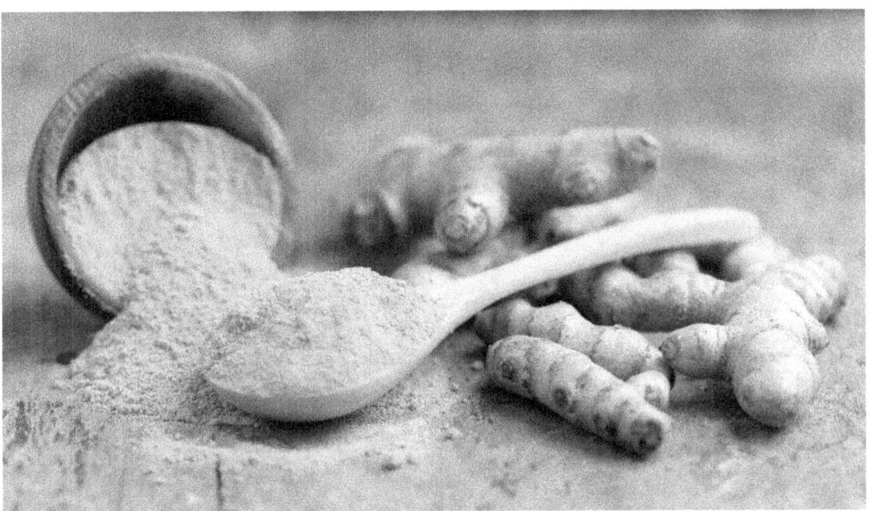

Turmeric is a bright yellow spice with a warm, slightly bitter taste. It is commonly used in curries and has anti-inflammatory properties.

Cayenne Pepper (Capsicum annuum)

Cayenne pepper is a hot chili pepper variety. It adds heat and spice to dishes and is often used in spicy foods, sauces, and seasonings.

Aloe Vera (Aloe vera)

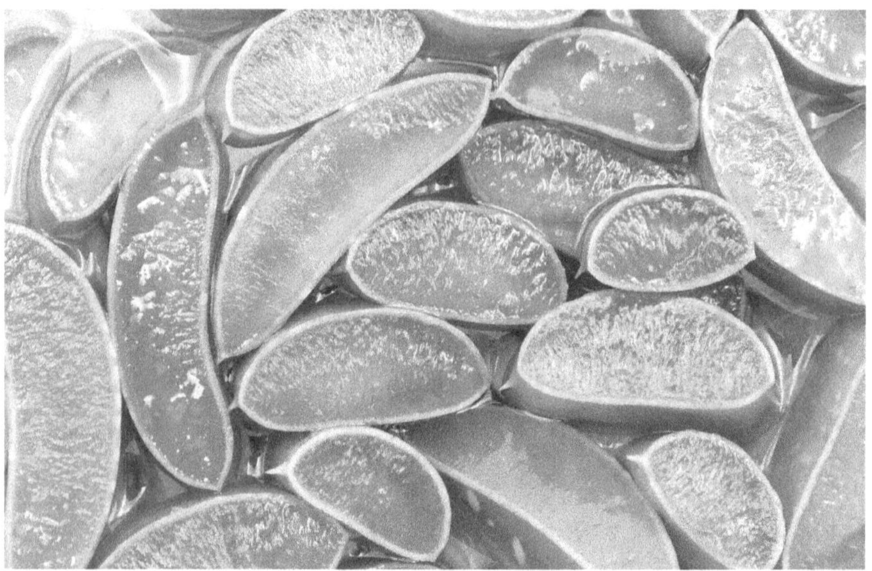

Aloe vera is a succulent plant known for its gel, which is used topically for skincare and sunburn relief. It is also consumed for potential internal health benefits.

These herbs and spices are not only valued for their flavors but also for their potential medicinal and wellness properties in various traditional and alternative medicine practices.

Medicinal plants...

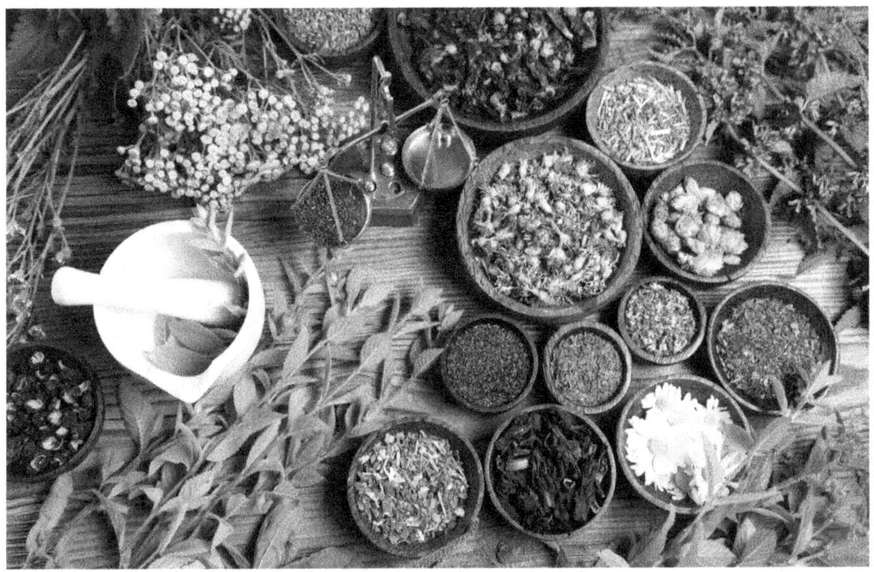

Herbs have always played a crucial role in human health and well-being. Used for their medicinal properties, herbs offer a wide range of benefits, from stress management to fortifying the immune system. In this chapter, we will explore the therapeutic power of some particularly well-known herbs.

Chamomile

Used for its calming and anti-inflammatory properties, chamomile is often employed in the treatment of allergies and as a remedy for relaxation.

Echinacea

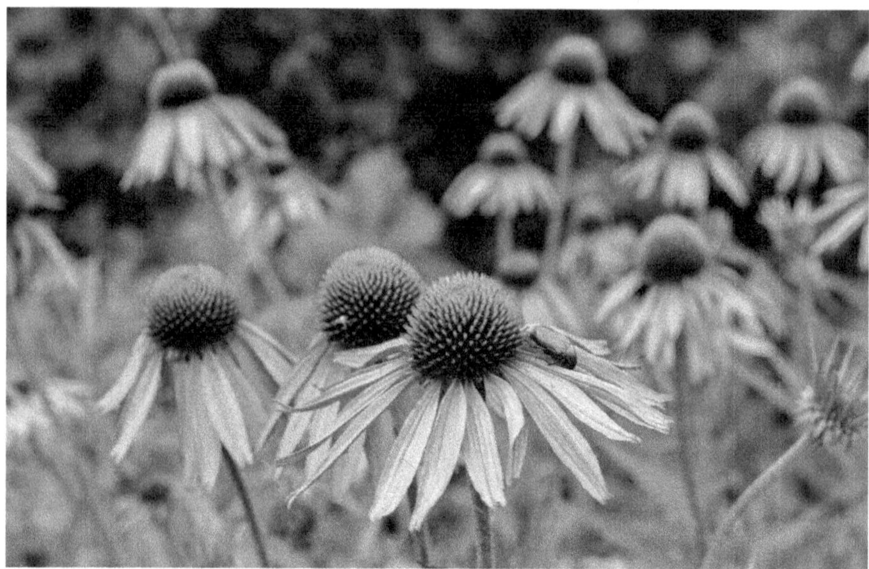

Its reputation for strengthening the immune system is well-known, making echinacea a valuable ally in disease prevention and facing periods of physical stress.

Ginseng

Known to increase energy and improve concentration, ginseng is often used as a natural tonic to combat fatigue and enhance cognitive performance.

Turmeric

Celebrated for its antioxidant and anti-inflammatory properties, turmeric is an ally in promoting joint health and managing inflammation.

Cayenne Pepper

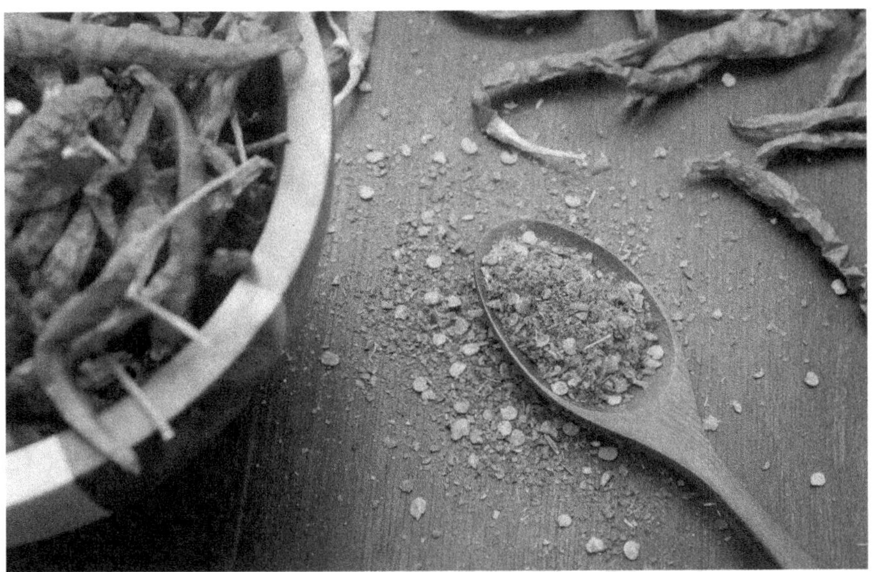

Used for pain relief and to improve circulation, cayenne pepper is a spice that can help reduce inflammation and promote cardiovascular well-being.

Ginger

Known for its anti-nausea and digestive properties, ginger is often recommended to alleviate gastrointestinal disorders and improve digestion.

Sage

Often used to treat respiratory and digestive system disorders, sage has properties that can contribute to the well-being of these areas.

Lavender

Used for its calming properties and to promote sleep, lavender is an herb with a pleasantly aromatic profile that offers relaxation benefits.

Valerian

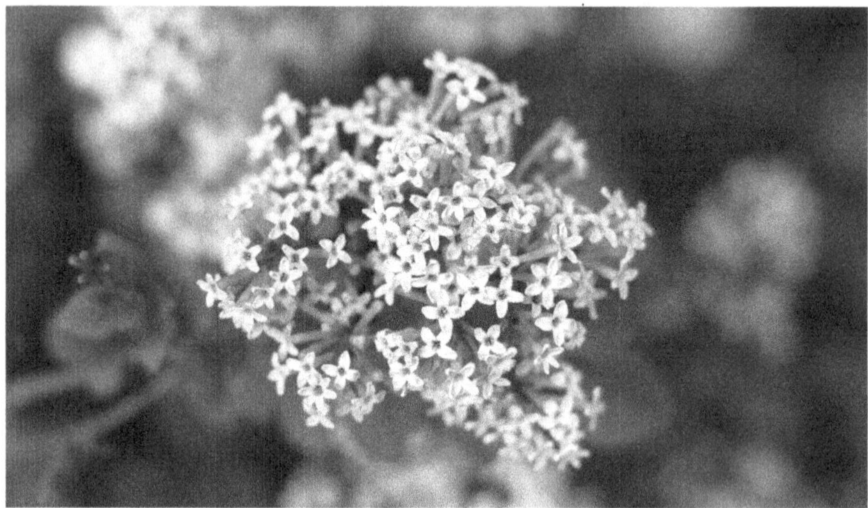

Known for its sedative properties, valerian is often used to help combat insomnia and improve sleep quality.

Aloe Vera

Used to soothe irritated skin and for the treatment of minor burns, aloe vera is a natural remedy for skincare.

"The Therapeutic Power of Herbs"

- **Hawthorn:** Beneficial for the heart.
- **St. John's Wort:** Used against burns.
- **Licorice:** Beneficial for the stomach.
- **Ginkgo Biloba:** Aids concentration.

- **Devil's Claw:** Useful against muscle and joint pain.
- **Calendula:** Applied for reddened skin.
- **Thyme:** Beneficial for the respiratory system.
- **Propolis:** For throat protection.
- **Mallow:** Promotes bowel regularity.
- **Nettle-Ginger:** Relieves joint pain.
- **Elderflower-Onion:** Used for flu grog.
- **Lavender-Hawthorn:** Used for anxiety (calming herbs).
- **Rosemary and Licorice Root:** Used for allergies.
- **Verbena-Lemon Balm-Valerian-Passionflower:** Used for insomnia.
- **Dandelion-Milk Thistle-Cumin and Mint:** Used for various beneficial purposes.
- **Peppermint-Pine Nut-Sweet Licorice:** Used to facilitate digestion.
- **St. John's Wort (Oil)-Witch Hazel (Leaves)-Aloe:** Used for burns.

These herbs not only enrich the culinary world but also serve as valuable resources to promote health and well-being naturally. Knowledge and conscious use of these herbs can contribute to a holistic approach to health maintenance.

Thanks for reading my book
I worked quite a bit on this manuscript
I kindly ask you to help me publish
a positive review

Conclusion

In this exploration through the pages of this book on medicinal herbs, we have delved into a world rich in tradition, wisdom, and potential health benefits. Herbs, with their unique properties, not only offer a sensory experience in the kitchen but also a treasure trove of potential natural remedies.

We've learned that chamomile can soothe not just tea cups but also storms of stress and inflammation. Echinacea has taught us to fortify our body's defenses, while ginseng has shown us the power of natural energy and concentration. Turmeric, with its vibrant colors, has guided us into the realm of antioxidants and the fight against inflammation.

From kitchens to herbal apothecaries, we've discovered that herbs are not just ingredients but valuable allies for our health. Cayenne pepper has invited us to experience healing warmth, while ginger has taken us down paths of liberated nausea and eased digestion.

The wisdom of sage has guided us through the trails of the respiratory and digestive systems, while the gentleness of lavender has enveloped us in a nighttime tranquility embrace. Valerian, with its sweet sedative melody, has offered us serene and restorative sleep, while aloe vera has soothed us with its therapeutic freshness.

We've explored the heart with hawthorn, challenged burns with St. John's Wort, and pampered the stomach with the sweetness of licorice. Ginkgo Biloba has accompanied us in the pursuit of concentration, while Devil's Claw has cradled our muscles and joints in a comforting relief.

Calendula has painted our world with a reassuring orange, alleviating reddened skin, while thyme has opened our respiratory pathways with its invigorating aroma. Propolis has acted as a guardian of the throat, while mallow has reminded us of the importance of regular bowel function.

The beauty of hawthorn has lulled us into relaxation, while nettle-ginger has eased joint pains, demonstrating that nature offers solutions for every season of life.

With the gentle touch of elderflower and onion, we faced the flu with a healing grog, while the combination of lavender and hawthorn guided us through the waves of anxiety.

With rosemary and licorice root, we confronted allergies, while verbena, lemon balm, valerian, and passionflower led us to deep and rejuvenating sleep.

Dandelion, milk thistle, cumin, and mint showed us the way to balanced health, while peppermint, pine nut, and sweet licorice played a melody of digestive facilitation.

With St. John's Wort (oil), witch hazel (leaves), and aloe, we healed burns and celebrated the healing power of plants.

In this journey, we experienced the blend of tradition and science, ancient and modern, the wisdom of herbs, and our commitment to health. Herbs, with their variety and versatility, invite us to integrate them into our daily lives to promote balanced well-being.

Let's always remember to consult qualified experts before undertaking any herbal regimen, recognizing that nature, with its herbs, offers us not just a treasure of health but also a responsibility in the conscious use of these precious resources.

May this book be a companion in discovery and reflection, inspiring us to forge a deeper connection with the world of herbs and encouraging us to explore the paths of health in harmony with nature. May our journey with herbs continue to bloom, just like the potential for well-being they offer.

www.ingramcontent.com/pod-product-compliance
Lightning Source LLC
Chambersburg PA
CBHW061059250726
48653CB00001B/466